I0658138

STORM DANCING

BY

MAC CUSITER

STORM DANCING

All rights reserved © 2016 by Mac Cusiter

No part of this book may be reproduced or transmitted in any form or by any means, graphic, electronic, or mechanical, including photocopying, recording, taping, or by any information storage retrieval system without the written permission of the author.

This book is a work of fiction. Names, characters, places, and incidents are products of the author's imagination or are used fictitiously. Any resemblance to actual events or locales or persons, living or dead, is entirely coincidental.

Cover Design: Mac Cusiter
Cover model © Elena Shchipkova | Dreamstime.com
Back Cover Design: Mac Cusiter
Storm image © Depositphotos-5-1968149_1-2015

Gurumbi Publishing
ISBN: 978-0-9941582-1-5

Printed in the United States of America

To my beloved wife Val for her perennial love and patience

The author would also like to thank Jane Flower for her enthusiastic encouragement. My sincere thanks to Heather Stootman, John Tesseyman and Robyn Claydon for their meticulous care in proofreading this manuscript

STORM DANCING

Chapter 1

The weather report was most unwelcome. "Hot with the possibility of afternoon showers, turning to rain later on in the evening. Another boost for retailers as shoppers seek the air conditioned comfort of department stores in the pre-Christmas rush."

So said Mike Jarvis with the omniscience every weatherman displays at the end of the evening news before the Sports Report. It was the twelfth of December, and Sydney had sweltered in forty degrees Celsius and sixty percent humidity for the last three days. "Unseasonable," someone from the Bureau had said, considering the fact that the heat wave had followed on from a pleasant fortnight of temperatures in the low twenties. No doubt the unpleasant thought of spending another tiring day at home, sweating it out to the sound of an ineffective little window rattling cooler, prompted the large crowds which filled the shopping malls from early that morning. Intent on staying there as long as possible, they spent their money with more than usual care and less than usual impulsiveness. Sales assistants found themselves being asked questions about their products they had long since forgotten the answers to, if they had ever known them.

Other assistants, who were wiser than those rushing to find the answers to questions their enquirers were not the slightest bit interested in, simply talked about the weather. Wasn't it stinking hot, and how nice it was to find a cool place. Did they know that the store had a very nice cafeteria on level three which served good wines with lunch at very reasonable prices? A short description of the food usually saw the customer making a bee-line for the cafeteria, desperate for a cup of tea or something a little more in keeping with the Christmas spirit, whatever that was.

By mid-morning the Bureau of Meteorology had revised its previous forecast to a strong wind warning with rain in the evening, heavy at times. The thousands of shoppers, drowned in the sounds of Jingle Bells and cash registers wouldn't have heard it even it had been broadcast to them – which it wasn't. Successive bulletins, upgrading the forecast to gale force winds with heavy rain and the possibility of local flooding passed them by as well. The utterly black skies over Sydney around four o'clock that afternoon were only noticed by those who had spent the day at home. They turned off their window rattlers and opened their homes to let the cooler air flood in. Most of those hadn't heard the forecast either, or if they had they probably welcomed it. Relief at last! Time to bring in the washing.

The first powerful gust of the storm struck at five fifteen, just as many of the shoppers were heading home after a comfortable if tiring day. A short time later traffic had ground to a halt, trains had stopped running, and in most suburbs the electricity supply had failed as well. Those commuters unfortunate to be stuffed like sardines into trains now dark and powerless, sweltered in conditions they had spent the whole day successfully avoiding. Those walking along the streets found they had to grab hold of something to avoid being bowled over by the force of the wind and tumbled into the torrent of water which had taken the place of the footpath.

Serious injuries increased by the minute, and the State Emergency Service was soon pushed to the limit of its capabilities. There were trees down on roads, railway lines and houses, people stranded in cars with rising water around them, and houses unroofed. In Cabramatta, the residents of a caravan park had to be evacuated before their vans bobbed away like boats in the torrent. Around six o'clock a block of units in Westmead partially collapsed because its foundations had been undermined by floodwaters. People were being rescued from upper storey windows by a determined and courageous fire brigade, whose officers could barely climb the ladders they had erected to provide the necessary escape.

In Sydney's northern suburbs the fury of the storm was perhaps a little less, but by six thirty the Pacific Highway was cut by fallen trees in three places. Hornsby Shopping Mall had lost the semicircular roof above its picture theatres, necessitating the evacuation of a sizeable crowd who had escaped into entertainment rather than face the grim realities of the world outside. Reality has its way of making its presence felt, however.

At seven o'clock the Premier called out the Army Reserve to assist the SES in its operations, which was politically correct but practically useless as all the phone lines to SES headquarters were jammed solid. Huge seas whipped up by the cyclonic winds were pounding the coast, and several homes on the northern beaches had completely disappeared along with the roads that led to them.

✳ ✳ ✳

At five o'clock, Joel Streetman and Jodie O'Connor, television hosts of The Morning Show, had been ordered out of their warm office where they were preparing tomorrow's offering for a panting public to go cover the coming storm drama. George, technician and general assistant, had been conscripted as their driver, all the others being unavailable. George didn't like driving the large outside broadcast van at the best of times, and this was certainly not one of those. They left the studio at ten past five and headed into the afternoon commuter traffic. The sky was black as midnight, the street lamps beginning to glow pinkish yellow as they do when they have just been turned on. George veered off Epping Road into quieter streets as soon as he could, and managed to reach Boronia Park before the first gust almost pushed him into the oncoming traffic.

Turning off into an even quieter street, he climbed up the rise until he had a clear view towards the city and surrounding suburbs. He switched on the satellite dish hydraulics and manoeuvred until he had a good signal. Unfortunately their vantage point also meant the satellite dish caught the wind like a sail, and soon the van was rocking back and forth in a most alarming manner. Now came the rain, reducing visibility to the point where George deeply regretted his choice of location. They could have seen more going through a car wash. He thought of trying to move the van down the hill, but decided the attempt would result in catastrophe. They pushed a camera up against the glass of the window in the side, locked its legs and gaff taped them to anything solid.

For all of ten minutes it had sent back pictures of the elemental fury and horizontal driving rain, illuminated by a local street lamp whose gooseneck was bending in the wind. Then the lamp went out, and all that remained was the weird blue splatter of the rain against the window every time the lightning flashed. Fearing their watching public would soon lose interest in such intermittent abstract art, the producer had told Joel and Jodie to send them something entertaining or return to the studio. George had refused point blank to move the van, so now Joel and Jodie were engaged in ad-lib banter in front of the camera, which their professional training and razor sharp wit enabled them to do for hours.

"That rain is really wet," Jodie said with her I'm-taking-you–into-my-confidence sort of voice. "I opened the window just a crack for a second ago and now I'm soaking."

"You're kinda sexy when you're all wet, Jodie," Joel said, eyeballing Jodie's soaking T shirt in a meaningful manner.

"I have this theory that storms make men think of sex," Jodie countered, facing deliberately into the camera. "Do you feel that way, viewers? SMS to the number on the bottom of your screens."

Not to be outdone, Joel progressed the theme. "I knew a girl who said she always had the best sex during a storm. Kinda romantic, isn't it? Perhaps the viewers would like to tell us if they've ever done it while the thunder rolled outside. Call the number on the bottom of your screen."

"Is that why you keep grabbing on to my arse every time the van tips over with the wind, Joel?"

"I do not," Joel retorted. "Close that shot in a bit, George. But speaking about arses in general, it's about time somebody kicked the Weather Bureau's. They really stuffed up this time, didn't they Jodie?"

"They sure did," Jodie agreed. "'Bout time they learnt to read all those dials and wind things. What do you call those wind things, Joel?"

The fact that there wasn't a working television set within the whole metropolitan area was at least one merciful blessing of the storm.

❋ ❋ ❋

Police Sergeants Daniel Lucas and his mate Brian Craig had been heading out west from Epping in their patrol car when the storm struck. Both young men, they had graduated from the Police Academy several years ago, and enjoyed working together. Within five minutes a tree had come down on a house in North Rocks and the owner had dialled triple zero, his wife was injured. SES were pushed beyond capacity, so the two policemen had been assigned the task. Arriving a few minutes later, they battled the torrential rain up to the splintered front door. A branch of the huge gum which had crushed the family car as well as the side of the house protruded into the hallway. They found the husband in shock and his wife lying in the bedroom, a nasty gash on her head and an obviously broken arm.

"She was in the family room when the ceiling collapsed," the husband said, pale and decidedly shaky. "Lucky to be alive. Have you seen our family room? It's just a pile of matchwood."

The woman was disorientated and her speech was slurred. Daniel fought his way back to the police car and radioed the situation. All ambulances were deployed, and if the woman was in need of critical care they should take her to Westmead Hospital themselves. It was no easy task to get her into the vehicle, what with the wind and the driving rain, and a husband who ought to have had medical attention himself. Eventually they managed it, and set off under siren down North Rocks Road, but the tropical deluge reduced visibility to almost zero. Just before the junction with Windsor Road they found Hunts Creek already over the bridge as it thundered towards the Parramatta River. It wouldn't be long before the junction was impassable.

Brian, who was driving, gritted his teeth and edged the car through the swirling torrent, feeling it slide from side to side in the current. He was a good driver, and that night he needed to be. Ten minutes later they arrived at Westmead Emergency to find the place already crowded. Half an hour later the woman was admitted, and the two police officers, who were drenched to the skin, decided a coffee from the hospital cafeteria was required for medicinal purposes before they fought their way back to the car.

It was barely five thirty on that summer evening when the power went down. Emergency lighting flickered on in the wards, dimmed, then flickered off again. Casualty was left in pitch darkness with people tripping over each other as they sought some source of light. Somewhere in the darkness a woman screamed, then another, until Daniel found it necessary to bellow for calm at the top of his voice, which rather detracted from his request. Nurses arrived bearing torches, followed by the Registrar who announced the hospital's emergency lighting plant had failed, but people were working on the problem. Actually they were trying to contact the service personnel who would no doubt work on the problem when they got there, but the Registrar thought it expedient to leave this complication out of his announcement. Daniel and Brian assisted where they could, preferring the gloom of Emergency to the soaking darkness which lay beyond it.

On the wards the situation was no better. Nurses ran helter-skelter from one crisis to another, their torches slowly becoming dimmer and less effective with every passing minute. By now Emergency was crammed to the gunnels with injured people, and triage had extended to the early hours of the morning, even for severe cases. Every doctor on duty was attempting to treat the ever increasing number of people, under conditions which resembled an army hospital on the front line.

Had they known it, the conditions at Royal North Shore and Liverpool hospitals were just as bad, although North Shore was running on its own generators. At least the staff could see where they were going, and doctors could use the operating theatres.

Storm Dancing

By half past eight the wind had died, and the torrential rain hissing down had lessened. Daniel decided they should make a break for the car to report in. Finding the car without any form of lighting was a far from easy task, and they bumped into several other vehicles before they found their own in the pitch black soaking night. The radio traffic was heavy and continuous. Daniel reported in. There was a triple zero call from a woman in Telopea, if they could get over Hunts Creek. If not, could they radio the condition of the road to HQ. Brian started the engine and they began to move slowly, turning right out of Emergency into Mons Road and heading towards the Cumberland Highway. Not far from the hospital Mons road crossed over Toongabbie Creek, by this stage running in a concrete water channel some six metres high and twenty wide. On either side, steep grassy banks opened out into public parkland further downstream. The bridge was just up ahead, or at least it had been when they arrived. With any luck it would still there and not under a metre of foaming water.

Suddenly Brian slewed the car to a stop, staring out the window as if his eyes were playing tricks on him. "What the blazes is that?" he yelled.

Caught in the glare of the headlights was a teenage girl, her face turned upward into the rain, eyes shut, mouth open. She was moving along the footpath by the creek in a bizarre twirling motion, her hands outstretched as if she was engaged in a strange dance, her wet, curly hair flapping from side to side across her face in time with the odd movement. She was dressed in a sodden white hospital gown, barely caught together by the one remaining tie across her back. Butt naked and bare footed she danced along in this manner oblivious of the headlights illuminating her for all the world to see. Suddenly she froze, her head jerked upright, and a pair of large terrified eyes turned into the glaring light. Her mouth opened in a scream they could hear inside the car, and twirling around round frantically, she tripped over her own feet and rolled out of sight down the embankment towards the surging swollen water.

In one movement Daniel snatched a torch from the glove box, opened the door and pelted along the path to the place where the girl had fallen. Shining the torch down toward the water he found her, impossibly dangling like a dead thing over the raging stream. Her thigh had caught

7

in a ditch carved by the water pouring down the grassy slope. It was a precarious position, not long to last. Her face was almost touching the foaming water, her arms already dragging in the surging current.

Daniel knew if he took his time to climb safely down the slope to where she lay, her body would have long been swept away and her life forfeited. Taking his own in his hands, he tobogganed on his backside down the slope towards her, praying the concrete lip on the channel would stop him, praying he wouldn't be the one to bump her off into oblivion.

He nearly did.

His foot found the channel lip just where the girl was wedged, and the impact of his landing dislodged her from her holding place. Daniel felt her slide, and grabbed her ankle with both hands as it flew past his face. He tried desperately to pull her back on top of him, all the time yelling for Brian to come quickly. Using every muscle he possessed, Daniel managed to drag the girl's ankle above his head, but whether he had succeeded in pulling her face away from the water he couldn't tell. Besides, his grip was slipping, and he dare not take a hand away in search for another body part to grab. The hospital gown was thrown over her head and acting as a sail in the stream which didn't help at all. Slowly he could feel her leg slipping from his grasp. Just as he despaired of saving her, he felt his partner – who had come down the slope with a great deal more care – take hold of her other leg and pull her to safety. Between the two of them they hauled the unconscious girl up the slope and carried her carefully back to the road and into the car. Brian switched on the light, and they took their second good look at the mud bespattered figure lying silent on the back seat.

"That was close." Daniel shook his head, "poor kid can't be more than eighteen – if she's that."

"Where did she come from?" Brian said, trying to wrap the muddy sodden garment around the girl's naked thighs.

"Westmead psych ward," Daniel suggested. "Remember the way she was moving when we spotted her? Better get her back, poor kid."

Just then the street lights came on.

They drove back to the hospital under siren, and parked close to the Emergency entrance. Leaving Brian to keep an eye on the girl, Daniel went into Casualty. He reflected that the lights glaring down from the ceiling accentuated the degree of human suffering crammed into the room. The darkness had been better. He walked to the counter and interrupted one of the triage nurses who looked as though she was going to commit murder with her bare hands any second. "Sorry to interrupt. We have one of your patients unconscious in the police car outside."

"Go and see Betty over there." The woman barked, hardly turning her head.

Daniel went over to see Betty and repeated this simple statement of fact.

Betty actually glanced up from the pile of paperwork strewn all over her desk, but her expression wasn't much different from that of the triage sister. "You'll have to see the Registrar. He's in there." She pointed with her hand rather abstractedly in the direction of the corridor leading to the wards.

Daniel, feeling this was going to be a far from simple task, followed her direction, and after a lot of questioning and being directed here and there, actually found the gentleman in his office typing numbers into a computer terminal. The long evening had taken its toll on him too.

"Yes?" The Registrar snapped at Daniel as he turned around.

"I've got one of your patients in the car," Daniel explained again. "Psych case, possibly. Unconscious. Found wandering a short distance away. Don't know if it's serious. Probably is. She almost drowned in Toongabbie Creek."

"Wait a minute." The Registrar turned back to his computer. More typing, pause, more typing. He turned around to face Daniel again.

"She's not one of ours. All our patients are present and correct. Losing them isn't the problem right now, it's where to put all the new ones."

"But she has to have come from here," Daniel protested. "The girl wasn't walking right. She couldn't have come far, not in the conditions out there. Check again."

The Registrar consciously assembled his face into the expression he wore when he was forced to deal with moronic members of the public when he wanted them to go away. "Officer, the first thing we did when the lights came on was check every ward. Each ward sister has reported in. We have no missing patients in any ward. If you want to waste your time like you're wasting mine you're welcome to check yourself."

"Then can you take her in emergency? She's unconscious, likely to have some sort of concussion."

"Have you seen emergency?" The Registrar's face had lost its suffering–with–patience expression. "Triage is up to next week. Sorry. You'll have to find somewhere else. Bye." He turned back to his computer screen and Daniel walked back to the car in a rather troubled frame of mind.

"Has there been any change, Brian?" he asked through the window.

"No. Do we take her in there now?" Brian reached for the door handle.

"No," Daniel sighed, "and they swear no patients are missing." Daniel swung himself onto the front passenger seat. "Has to be a mistake. Get on the radio, Brian, and see what you can do at North Shore or Concord or anywhere. We can't go around all night with an unconscious half-naked girl in the back of the car. I don't want her dying on us, especially when we both risked our necks to save her life."

Ten minutes on the radio was all it took to convince both officers that the very last place their charge was going to get medical help was the emergency department of any hospital in the Sydney Metropolitan Area.

Daniel sighed and rubbed his hand against his mud streaked forehead. "Can't leave the poor kid on the back seat all night. Any ideas?"

Storm Dancing

"I might have," Brian said. "My brother is a doctor at Cherrybrook. Damn good one. Married a Hungarian girl he met in Medical school called Basa. She's a cardiologist. Yeah, I know what you're thinking. I got the dumb genes. I'll phone them if you like. If we get his wife first I think we're screwed, but we might get lucky."

They got lucky. Hunts Creek bridge was still impassable, so they detoured down James Ruse Drive, took the Pennant Hills exit, and half an hour later Brian rang the bell on the surgery door. Andrew came out, said 'hello' to his brother and stared at the unconscious mud spattered child in Daniel's arms.

"Bring her in, quickly," he instructed. "Lay her down on the paper." Then calling out through the door, "Basa, the girl's here. Still unconscious." He turned to his brother: "Where did you find her?"

Both doctors were in the room while the story was retold. Basa nodded meaningfully towards her husband and advanced on the patient stretched out in muddy silence on the examination table.

Andrew ushered the police officers out of the room. "Would you like to stay for a cup of something, Brian? I'm sorry I didn't catch your mate's name."

"Daniel. No thanks, Andrew. We've probably got a long night to go. Thanks once again. We'll keep trying to find out where the kid comes from. Let you know as soon as we hear anything. No point in trying to get her into hospital casualty. It's like a war zone out there."

The men walked out of the house and Andrew went back to join his wife in the surgery. By the time he arrived the muddy hospital gown was on the floor, and Basa was sponging some of the mud away from the girl's face. There were a few superficial scratches here and there, but nothing to indicate a serious blow. Andrew with his usual care began to check vital signs, took her blood pressure – normal, temperature – normal. He listened to her heart and chest. He lifted each eyelid to find both eyes rolled towards the back of her head, and then began to examine other parts of her body. He fished a towel out of the cupboard, threw it into the sink, turned on the tap and added disinfectant to the water. Now to wash the mud off the rest of the girl in case some injury was hiding under it.

He turned to his wife who was running her fingers over the patient's head. "Found any wounds of significance?"

"Not yet.. wait... There's a lump here. I can feel it with my fingers. Let's see."

Running her fingers through the curly strands of hair, Basa began to part it gently away from the scalp to reveal a small cut in the middle of a somewhat larger lump. "This could have knocked her out," she said frowning, "but it doesn't seem all that serious to me. I'll clean it up and put....and put... Andrew, stop what you're doing and look at this."

"What's up? Found the injury site? Hello, now that's odd. Follow it around."

Both doctors began parting the girl's hair across the top of her head, then around the sides, occasionally glancing at one another.

Finally Andrew spoke softly as if to himself. "There's lots of them, all in parallel."

Basa nodded. "Beautiful work. No two bob plastic surgeon did that."

"But why?" Andrew asked. "I'd say the girl has had extensive—"

"Cranial surgery," Basa interrupted. "That's what I think. Your brother was searching in the wrong hospital department. He should have tried the neurological ward. Andrew, wash the rest of that mud off her, will you?"

"What do you expect to find? Hello, she didn't get that falling down the hill."

STORM DANCING

The disappearing mud had revealed a small scar above the girl's left breast. Basa examined it closely. "Possibly the site of an old central line. Wash the mud off her legs."

Andrew washed the mud off her right one, and then began the same process with her left. On her left thigh another scar became visible.

"Surely…" Andrew said, shaking his head, "another central line site, and this one has only just been closed. You can still see the stitches. Less than twenty four hours I'd say."

"Central line," Basa said thoughtfully. "She's been fed through a central line. Andrew, get me a spatula, will you?" She gently separated the girl's legs, and taking the spatula from her husband's hand, carefully parted her labia. "Urethral catheterisation, long term. Some peripheral scarring and traces of infection. Concur?"

"No doubt of it," Andrew agreed. "But why? The cranial scarring is completely healed. Why was she on total parenteral nutrition? Must be some other problem… Vitals are all normal."

"Bowel blockage?" Basa queried. "Check her peristalsis."

Andrew fetched his stethoscope and ran the instrument over the girl's stomach. "Perfectly normal, I'd say, consistent with a patient who has gone to sleep. These small scars around her stomach area, hardly visible. What do you think?"

"Have no idea. There must be other marks. She was being treated for something, Andrew. That was a hospital gown she was wearing. The child walked out of a hospital ward, and it wasn't because she'd just had cranial surgery."

For the next ten minutes both doctors examined the patient in minute detail, turning her over on one side, then the other. There was not a trace of any other injury, any other surgery.

"Long term catheterisation, long term feeding. That level of incapacity suggests coma, but those cranial scars have completely healed. No neurosurgeon would sustain a coma patient for years. They'd diagnose brain death and take her off life support," Basa said, re-examining the girl's head.

"Unless she had a relapse," Andrew frowned. "Perhaps a tumour on the brain? That's a horrible possibility. She has the surgery, she goes home, and a year or so later it comes back and they have to hospitalise her. She slips into a coma again. The surgeons realise it's the end and take the central line out, leave her to die."

"And die she would," Basa said. "No patient in that condition gets up and walks out of the ward by herself."

"But she wasn't at all normal, was she? Head up into the rain, twisting about trying to walk. I think the tumour theory is probably correct. Poor little girl." Andrew threw the dirty towel back into the sink. "But no, no, hang on. A terminal patient disappears from a neurological ward and nobody notices? I just don't believe anyone could be so careless, even given the storm and all."

"Unless they moved her into palliative care somewhere," Basa said sadly. "The storm woke her up – against all odds - and she wandered out, not really knowing what was happening. Then the fall causes bleeding around the tumour, and she goes back into a coma. Probably won't last the night." She sighed heavily. "In the morning her family will come to the hospital to say good-bye, and all hell will break loose."

"Then we should hear from Brian early tomorrow," Andrew said, taking a fresh towel from the cupboard, his face troubled. "What now? We can hardly leave the child to die on our examination table."

Their morbid thoughts were suddenly interrupted. The dying child gave a loud grunt and turned herself over, drew her legs up towards her stomach and lay still again. Basa and Andrew practically jumped off the floor.

"She's just asleep! For goodness sake, how is that possible?" Andrew exclaimed.

"She may not be, Andrew," Basa said sadly. "The tumour might be pressing on a motor area. We don't have an EEG machine here or we could tell. No, I think we're right. The poor child has come from palliative care. Such a tragedy, so young. She can't be more than seventeen or eighteen. Wash the rest of that mud off and we'll put her in the spare room. I'll prepare a sedative injection in case she wakes up distressed. Take my word for it, someone is probably searching high and low for her right now. Come on, let's try to make her clean and comfy." Basa took another washer from the cupboard. "I've just had an idea. Most hospital gowns have the name of the hospital on them. Check that, will you darling?"

Andrew lifted the sodden gown off the floor and turned it carefully round in his hands until he had examined it all. "Nothing on this one. I'll chuck it in the bin. That's it, now hand me that washer with the antiseptic, thanks."

It took no more than ten minutes for them to finish washing the girl down. The disappearing mud revealed some more scratches, some of which they treated with antiseptic, but most of them were superficial. Basa, completing her preparations, came over and towelled the girl gently dry, then Andrew lifted her as carefully and smoothly as he could off the table, out of the surgery door, down the corridor and onto the bed in the spare room. If she was just asleep this would not be the best time for her to wake up and find herself being carried naked in a strange man's arms.

While Andrew covered her up with a sheet and a doona, Basa fetched a baby monitor out of the cupboard and set it up on the bedside table. She paused, then went out of the room and returned with a dressing gown, which she placed folded on the end of the bed. "I know it's being silly, but... just in case she wakes up again," Basa said quietly. "If she stirs we'll hear her. Now, my love, it's time for bed. This has been quite an evening with the storm and all. I'm tired. It will be another long day tomorrow, and you have patients arriving at nine."

Andrew took his wife in his arms and kissed her. "Right as usual my Beauty. What would I do without you?"

With those endearing words they headed down the corridor to bed.

In the early hours of the morning Basa woke up. Andrew was breathing heavily beside her, and not wishing to wake him she turned over as smoothly as she could to see the time faintly displayed on their bedside alarm clock. Four thirty. Lightning still flashed behind the curtains and distant thunder boomed, reminding her the storm had not yet run its course of destruction, but the storm hadn't woken her up. It was the dream. She was alone in the surgery, staring at the silent, naked figure on the examination table, thinking how sad it was that a young girl should suffer from a terminal brain tumour. Something was troubling her, and she didn't know what it was. She came closer to repeat her observations. Suddenly the girl sat bolt upright and screamed in a very loud voice,

"You're wrong, you're wrong!"

That's what woke her up. Even now she could feel herself shaking from the nightmare. She carefully rolled over and tried to go back to sleep, but the strange girl's words were still echoing in her head. She had missed something. Her subconscious mind was telling her what her conscious mind had not been able to see. But what? She thought back over the evidence. The girl's vital signs were normal, there were only superficial injuries and those scars on her chest and thigh – and suddenly she saw the fallacy in the argument.

Time.

They had even talked about it, but somehow they had lost the thread…the girl had moved suddenly and startled them, yes, that's what had happened. Time. In hospital, especially in a neurological ward, a carefully tended central line could last for twelve months, probably longer. This girl had been the recipient of two, one after the other. Any brain tumour, sufficiently advanced to reduce her to that level of dependence, would have killed her in days, weeks at most. Some other severe problem had to be the cause, but then the same argument applied. She would be dead in weeks, not months, not years. And then, why remove the line? Surely that meant they had given up hope. Or she had recovered. But then, if she had recovered, why didn't she wake up with all the activity going on around her? No one stays asleep through the rigorous examination she and Andrew had subjected her to.

More questions than answers, but the brain tumour theory was dead on the floor. Perhaps she had come from a psychiatric ward and not palliative care, but then why the central line? Her brain tumour had been excised, but it had left her with severe mental retardation, so much so she couldn't even feed herself? That would explain it, perhaps.

Either way, Basa was glad the girl was going in the morning. Reaching out she grabbed the baby monitor, and turning up the volume, held it next to her ear. The girl was breathing normally, regularly. She gave a little grunt and sounds of doona rustling came over the monitor followed by regular slow breathing again. So normal, so completely bizarre.

CHAPTER 2

The Craig household rose at five thirty every morning, even in the school holidays. Father had to be in the surgery by eight when Annette his secretary arrived, and Mother was due out half an hour earlier. Peter, their seventeen year old, caught the bus to Pennant Hills High School around the same time. Ellen, their ten year old Surprise and Delight, would be accompanied over the road by Annette to be minded by Sharon until primary school started at nine. The early start meant the family could spend a guaranteed quality hour together around the breakfast table each day. Both parents being doctors, quality time was not something the family were guaranteed of in the evenings. Basa was often called out to some emergency, and sometimes didn't get home until the small hours. Andrew's patients were more or less local, but he was one of those doctors who still made house calls which could come at any time. Through years of experience they had found the hour at which medical emergencies were at their lowest ebb – six o'clock in the morning. Very rarely had their family time been interrupted, and it was to the credit of every member of the household that they valued it so highly.

The breakfast routine was always the same. Basa would arrive first and begin cooking omelettes for herself and Andrew, a boiled egg each for Peter and Ellen.

Peter would stagger in next, half asleep and uncommunicative, drag out the toaster and start cooking toast. Ellen would bounce into the room, wide awake on full power and begin setting the table. Andrew was last to arrive. He would go over to the stove and give Basa a good morning kiss, hug Ellen as she made another trip to collect utensils from the dishwasher, sit down at the table opposite Peter and say 'good morning' to him. Peter was by now at the grunting stage, but after a juice and his egg he would turn into the good natured lad he was, even though getting words out of him took a lot of effort at any time.

Ellen, on the other hand, was difficult to switch off.

Every inch a little girl, nobody had taught her what to do with her eyes and her bewitching smile, how to move every muscle of her body to make herself totally irresistible to her father. There were times her mother found herself taking note of the techniques she employed.

Before they had risen from their bed, Basa and Andrew had discussed whether they would tell their children about the sick girl in the spare room and decided to leave the news until after their family breakfast hour had run its course. Before turning on the stove, Basa had stolen quietly into her room and found her breathing steadily and showing not the slightest sign of returning to consciousness. Poor child, she thought again. What was the matter with her? She hoped Brian wouldn't ring or come to collect her before they finished breakfast.

Andrew and Ellen had already sat down at the table. Basa was cooking the second omelette. Peter retrieved the last piece of toast from the toaster, added it to the pile already on the plate, and brought the collection to the table. Sitting down, he picked up the boiled egg lying on his serviette, inserted in into the egg cup on his plate, and was about to execute the delicate operation of slicing off the top with his spoon. Ellen poured herself a large glass of milk from the jug on the table.

"Good morning, Peter." Andrew paused, waiting for the customary grunt which told him Peter had registered his early morning greeting. When it wasn't forthcoming he looked up from his omelette at the lad to find out why. Peter was sitting with his mouth open, his spoon poised in mid-slice, his eyes staring at some point in space behind his father's chair.

19

"Gosh!"

Peter's loud remark caused Ellen to glance up suddenly, and Basa to pause in the delicate operation of transferring her omelette from pan to plate. Ellen gave a loud infectious giggle, Basa put the pan down on the bench, and Andrew turned round to see what all the family was staring at. In the entrance to the hall stood a naked young woman, her eyes silently surveying the scene in front of her. If she was embarrassed by her nakedness or even aware of it she gave no sign at all. Her eyes flitted purposefully from one member of the family to the next. Peter, being a boy of all seventeen years, had seen naked girls before in the person of his sister, and naked women from the pages of certain magazines which his classmates kept private in their school bags. However he had never seen such an excellent example in the flesh before, and to say the sight held his attention was an understatement.

"Gosh!" He repeated, not quite as loudly this time.

"Young lady, would you please return to your room and put your dressing gown on," Basa commanded loudly. "Now!"

The naked girl turned to face her, tipped her head slightly to one side, paused as if she was considering the words addressed to her, then turned her attention back to the table. Her eyes lit up with joy. She gave what could have passed for a yelp of delight, and began to move forward in the strangest manner any of the family had ever seen. Instead of walking straight, her feet kept turning her around, almost tripping over themselves as they did. It would have been comical to watch were it not obvious that the owner of those feet did not want them to do what they seemed determined to keep doing. With every twist the girl was trying to control the turning motion. In the end her desire to move towards the table overcame her protest.

Eventually, as though some battle of wills had ended in defeat, she let her feet take her there however they wished, twirling her around and around faster and faster. Within arm's reach of the table she stopped, the entire Craig family staring at her in stupefied silence. Suddenly she snatched the egg that Peter was about to slice, and stuffed the whole lot

20

in her mouth. There were some crunching noises. A disgusted expression disfigured her face for a second, and then the egg – or rather the masticated remains of it – came out very much faster than it had gone in, distributing itself over the floor, the table and Peter himself in about equal portions.

"Gosh!" Peter uttered his third word for the morning.

The show wasn't done yet. Leaning over the table, the girl grabbed hold of the large milk jug, inverted it over her upturned mouth, and began gulping it down as though her life depended on emptying it. No doubt quite a lot of milk ended up down her throat, but an awful lot of it also streamed down her cheeks, splashed on the top of her breasts, and ran down her cleavage in a concentrated narrow stream, travelling smoothly downwards. It reached her tummy button and made a little whirlpool before completing its journey and plunging to the tiled floor in a white waterfall. The jug was almost empty when it became obvious to the family, staring incredulously at the spectacle, that the white waterfall had been joined by an even larger stream of a different colour. Basa said something loudly in Hungarian, and ran towards the surgery for the sedative injection she had prepared the night before, fearing worse was to come.

Ellen, possessed by a moment of that extraordinary insight and wisdom which any adult would be proud to own, got out of her chair and paddled through the growing puddle on the floor until she was standing beside the strange girl.

She held out both her hands towards her. "Come on, I'll show you where it is," she encouraged. "Let's *dance* there!"

The strange girl stared down at her as if she was trying to make sense of the gesture. All of a sudden she put down the empty jug on the table and extended her hands for Ellen to hold. Together they danced out of the room, turning round and round as they went down the hall towards the bathroom. Andrew, recovering from the shock of the last few minutes, got out of his chair and followed, telling Peter to stay where he was. He arrived at the bathroom door and stopped. Should he go in? Should he

21

respect the girl's privacy? Not if Ellen was having difficulties. He decided to listen outside.

After a short while Ellen's innocent little voice came floating out the door. "That's it. Wipe, wipe, wipe, drop. Your poo is a funny colour. Bend over. Here, more paper, wipe, wipe, wipe. Now we flush, see, like this."

"Wipe, wipe, wipe drop. Your poo is a funny colour." The strange girl's voice.

"That's right," Ellen giggled. "Can you say FLUSH?"

"Can you say flush?" The strange girl echoed Ellen's words. Both girls were laughing now, and although the older girl's pitch was slightly lower, the manner of both was identical.

"Now we wash hands," Ellen said in a mothering voice. "Turn the tap – not that much!" More laughter. "That's right. Now we use the soap. You've never done this, have you? Now wash, no, hands together, like me. That's it. Good girl, here's a towel."

"Good girl, here's a towel." The strange girl mimicked Ellen perfectly.

Andrew was struck by a sudden and irrational thought. No, surely, and yet... He turned around in time to see Basa barrelling down the hall, a naked syringe in her hand. He ran towards her, deliberately blocking her path. "I don't think we need to do that."

"What do you mean?" Basa snapped at him. "The child has acquired intracranial injury, severe intellectual impairment, disabled, incontinent, can't even walk properly, can't speak. She didn't escape from a hospital. She came from some sheltered workshop, and she's probably violent – that's why she got out. Andrew, step out of the way. Are you prepared to put our family at risk? A quick injection and you ring Brian. Tell him to check sheltered workshops."

"Does she look abnormal?" Andrew said gently.

"No," Basa barked. "Injury was acquired later on. Andrew!"

Andrew was still blocking her path. "She can talk, perfectly. She's echolalic." Andrew gently gripped Basa's injection wielding arm. "Could someone with the intellectual impairment you describe be capable of learning anything?"

Basa stared at Andrew as though he had lost his mind. Their daughter was in the bathroom with this girl, anything could happen. "Impossible. Why ask me what you know? Andrew, for the last time, move out of the way. Help me catch her when she collapses."

"Then why is she learning from Ellen how to go to the toilet?"

"What nonsense is this?" Basa jerked her arm free.

"Basa, indulge your stupid husband for ten minutes. If I'm wrong – and I admit it makes no sense – then give her the injection."

"What are you proposing we do, sit back until she pees on the lounge room carpet, picks up a knife and slashes someone?" Basa glared at her husband.

"Just watch her for a while, that's all I ask," Andrew said persuasively. "There's something very odd happening here."

Basa gave Andrew a furious stare, then glanced at her watch. She placed the safety cap on the syringe needle. "It's ten to seven. Don't play with the safety of my family on a whim, Andrew. Ten minutes, I sedate her, then you call Brian. Okay?"

"Okay. Here they come. Hide the syringe."

"Ten minutes, remember," Basa muttered under her breath. She turned to her daughter. "Ellen, take her into the bedroom and make her put on a dressing gown. There's one on the end of the bed."

Their patient appeared in the bathroom door holding Ellen's hands with both her own. The child made a determined effort to turn her in the direction of the bedroom, but her dancing partner gave a soft growl of protest, and being the stronger of the two, determined the direction. Back to the table they went to continue unfinished business. Andrew followed, with Basa muttering protests under her breath. If it hadn't been for the uncertainty precipitated by her dream, she would have stuck the needle in the girl as she passed.

Peter, his hands on the mop he was using to wipe the floor, stared at the duo twisting through the door in sheer disbelief. He grabbed the bucket and mop and retreated to the kitchen, watching his sister and the stranger as they went round and round towards the table. As a child he remembered reading a book about Wacky Wednesday. The degree of wackiness this morning left the book standing. Not that he minded. On the contrary, the morning had been most educational. Close to the table now, the stranger grabbed a piece of Ellen's toast and stuffed it in her mouth as though she hadn't eaten for a month.

She was about to grab the second piece but Ellen, predicting the move, had grabbed it first. Not to eat it, no, she had another idea. Holding the toast behind her she pushed the strange girl back towards a chair. "Sit down," she commanded. "You have to sit down for breakfast."

The strange girl stopped, tilted her head slightly as though she was trying to work out what Ellen had said. She surveyed the table to find it sadly devoid of further food, looked back at Ellen with her hand behind her back, and sat down.

Pulling up a chair near her, Ellen held out a piece of toast. "Here it is," she said in a very bossy voice, "when you've finished there's another piece."

The stranger took the toast from the plate where Ellen had placed it and stuffed it into her mouth. After some chewing noises she swallowed, turned back to Ellen and pointed to her empty plate.

"When you've finished there's another piece." The strange girl mimicked Ellen exactly.

"That's right, here," Ellen said, quite unaware of the girl's echolalia.

Proud of her controlling achievement she placed another piece on the plate. It disappeared like the first. "She's still hungry, Mum." Ellen turned to her mother. "Can you bring me something? See, she's got the idea now."

Basa stared at the girl for a full minute in silence, then returned to the kitchen for more food. Over the next ten minutes their naked guest managed to consume Basa's omelette, a slice of ham, two more pieces of toast, one with jam – great enjoyment – one with peanut butter – not so appreciated – and a large slice of cheese. Then the event which gave Basa's intellectual impairment theory its first challenging blow – a whole glass of milk, delivered carefully in small stages by Ellen who showed her how to put the cup to her lips and drink without spilling it everywhere. A further test was in order.

Basa went to the bedroom, picked up the dressing gown, and headed back to stand in front of the girl. "Put this on," She ordered.

"Put this on," the girl replied in exactly the same commanding voice. Ellen dissolved into giggles.

Basa handed the garment to the girl. She took it from her hand and began to turn it around in an aimless and somewhat disinterested fashion. She stuck one arm in an arm hole the wrong way round, tried to put the garment over her head, and finally, with a grunt of disgust which needed no interpretation, dropped the whole thing on the floor.

"Peter, turn you back, please," Basa called towards the kitchen.

Going over to a chair, Basa removed her own clothing and returned to the girl with the gown in her hand. "It goes on like this," she explained.

She put the gown on slowly and tied the cord around her waist. Then she untied it, took the gown off, and put it on again, finally handing the garment to the naked child. The strange girl smiled, and standing up, put the dressing gown on exactly as she had seen Basa do it.

"It goes on like this," she said, gave a little grunt to show how pleased she was with herself and sat down, staring meaningfully at her empty cup.

"Be damned," Basa muttered, returned to the chair and dressed. "You may turn around now Peter, and thank you. Andrew, what do you make of all this? Yes, Ellen, you can give her some more milk. The child seems incredibly thirsty."

"Which is why Brian found her with her face up in the storm," Andrew smiled to himself. "She was drinking the rain."

"Be damned again," Basa muttered. "You're thinking amnesia, aren't you? Well it won't work. She might have forgotten who she is, but to forget everything? No, no. How do you fit our observations of last night into the picture?"

"I have no idea," Andrew answered, "but the sheltered workshop theory won't fly either. I think we should discuss this by ourselves. The ten minutes is more than up and you have a big op this morning. You go, my Beauty, and I'll phone Brian as agreed. My receptionist might have to keep a bit of an eye on things here, but I'll manage."

"I'm not happy, Andrew," Basa said, frowning heavily. "The girl can't be stable. Anything could happen. For goodness sake take the kitchen knives into the surgery will you? Tell Brian to check sheltered workshops and the like. If anything happens, I want to know."

She came close and kissed him, gathered her shoes from the chair and walked out of the room. Andrew watched his seven year old teaching a girl at least twice her age to eat some custard with a spoon, much to the amusement of his son. He picked up the phone and called Brian.

A very tired voice answered him. "Andy, it's been one helluva night. That girl still unconscious? There's not a chance of a hospital admission anywhere in Sydney. That was some storm. Prime Minister has called it a national disaster. Seen the morning news?"

"No, and no, she isn't unconscious anymore. I take it you've checked the missing persons? No? Don't blame you. Just keep an eye out, will you? Could you check with sheltered workshops and the like? I'm going to ring the hospital. Are you going home soon? Good. Ciao."

Andrew wasn't the least bit surprised with the news. He never expected Brian to have done anything more than cope with the aftermath of the storm. If it hadn't been for his wife, he would never have rung him at all. Westmead hospital would be a different matter. If they couldn't spare an ambulance he would offer to take her there himself after his morning patients. He rang the number.

Half an hour later he put down the phone. He hadn't been surprised before, but he was now, astounded, rather. Not one patient was missing. He had described the girl, her condition, and indicated the ward from which she was most likely to have escaped. Then he had spoken to the sister in charge of that ward. He had contacted the nurse in charge of palliative care. He had a long and unpleasant conversation with a doctor in psychiatry.

Everyone said the same, only the way they said it changed the more he persisted. The last conversation with the director of patient care was far from friendly. Yes, they would let him know if any mentally deranged teenager had escaped from any ward in the last six months. Now would the good Doctor Craig please let them get on with the business of running a hospital? He had rung two sheltered workshops – which were nowhere near Westmead - with predictable results. No one fitted the girl's description, and no patients were missing. Why was he still asking? No, they couldn't help. They didn't cater for that level of disability. Had he thought of ringing psychiatric institutions who took permanent child patients?

Glancing out the window he saw his receptionist slide her car into her private parking space. Ten to eight. What had happened to the morning? Half an omelette and a cold cup of coffee had hardly prepared him for the twenty or so patients who came before lunch.

Annette, entering the house from the surgery, came into the room with a smile and a spring in her step. "Morning Andrew," she said. "What, still finishing breakfast? Hi Ellen, Peter. Who's the new girl? Cousin? What's her name?"

"Ah... yes, she's a new patient of mine... her name..." Andrew stammered.

The expression on her father's face instantly raised Ellen's protective instinct. "Storm," She piped up suddenly, smiling sweetly into the secretary's face. "I think it's a beautiful name, don't you?"

"Well, I've never met a "Storm" before,' Annette said, "but yes, it's a pretty name. Hello Storm."

The girl stared at the strange woman, smiled. "It's a pretty name. Hello Storm," she said.

Ellen, could see some urgent action was required. Her father seemed even more anxious than before. A sudden premonition crossed Ellen's perceptive little mind. This fascinating person was somehow in danger of being taken away. That was what was troubling her father. Ellen had no idea how Storm came to be in their home, but she knew the girl was helpless. She ran over to Annette, and taking her arm, turned her away from their guest, urging her towards the door. "She's got a really nasty contage-i-us throat infection," she confided softly. "That's why daddy's taking care of her. He'll have to drop in during the day for her medication. I didn't want you to catch it. We've all had injections."

Whatever Ellen lacked in age she more than made up for in imagination. Creative explaining, she called it, and her ability to craft fantasy had grown as quickly as her skill with the language she needed to create it. The big, sincere eyes just added to the convincing effect. Annette came with her willingly. The last thing she wanted was a nasty contagious throat infection.

"Annette," Andrew asked, "could you get my patient cards out? I'll be there in a jiffy. Thanks."

He waited until the woman had left the room then turned to his daughter, half in annoyance, half in admiration. "Ellen, how many times have I told you not to manufacture stories? Where did you dream that name from?"

"She came with the storm," Ellen said matter-of-factly. "It's a good name, don't you think? You know, Daddy, I don't think she has another name."

"Perhaps she just can't remember it," Andrew sighed. "Now Peter, I want a quiet word with you. Go on Ellen, but Storm can't have any more custard unless you want her to be sick all over the floor. Then it's you who has to clean up, not Peter. Oh… and you'd better take her to the toilet again. We don't have any nappies big enough."

He beckoned to his son, and the two of them left the room together. Sufficiently far into the lounge so as not to be overheard, he turned to Peter and spoke quietly. "Son, your father is very proud of the way you handled yourself this morning."

"That's okay, Dad," Peter grinned. "She's quite an … ah … shapely baby, isn't she?"

"She's very pretty, and she's also very sick. Mum and I don't know exactly what's wrong with her. That's the problem, we don't have a diagnosis, so we can't predict what will happen. There's a real possibility she might become unstable. If there are any indications you have to let me know. Immediately, even if I'm with a patient. If I've gone out, and push comes to shove there's an injection in the kitchen cupboard, top shelf with the glasses. If you give that to her – anywhere – she'll go to sleep. Only as a last resort. I want you to keep a close eye on her, and Ellen. You're in charge. Make sure Ellen is safe. I'm relying on you."

"What sort of disease has she got, Dad? She acts like a baby – except for the dancing thing."

"She might have some sort of mental illness, or her brain has been damaged, perhaps by a tumour. We think that's more likely. Perhaps she was born with brain damage, in which case you will have to be very careful. Your mother and I thought she was in a coma last night and didn't expect her to come out of it, so we didn't mention anything to you before breakfast. There may be some other explanation. Your mother thinks we're foolish to keep her here for more than five minutes. I'm not so sure. There's something about her which mystifies me, intrigues me as a doctor. If she shows the slightest trace of hostility, or we can't manage her, she's out of here."

"Another question, Dad. How come she's here at all? When did she get here?"

Andrew gave his son a condensed version of yesterday evening's events, watching the frown deepen on his forehead.

"Someone must be really worried by now," Peter said, frowning. "I can't understand why they haven't contacted the police."

"I'm sure they have," Andrew sighed, "but it's chaos out there. Uncle Brian has been on the go all night. Oh, and if he rings about Storm, come and get me too, will you. Have to go."

❋ ❋ ❋

The morning passed without further incident. Andrew returned at lunchtime for a progress report from Peter.

"It's all going well, Dad," Peter informed him. "There was a bit of an incident when Ellen, little bossy-boots, tried to teach Storm to walk properly. She got really frustrated and threw Ellen's iPod out the window. Ellen's been huffy ever since, and Storm's playing like a kid on her own in the family room. I've made you a sandwich. It's on the kitchen bench."

"Thanks Peter. I'm starving."

"Not like Storm, you're not," Peter laughed. "She found a packet of biscuits in the pantry, and, well, you know the rest. She might be a baby, but she knows how to ferret out food."

Peter returned to supervision duties and Andrew walked into the kitchen. He poured himself out a glass of cold filtered water from the 'fridge, and sat down to eat the sandwich which his son had so thoughtfully prepared. He had only just finished when Peter came back into the room.

"Dad, I think you should see this."

"Everything okay?"

"Yeah, Ellen's back in the family room and still a bit twitchy. Quick, before it's gone."

Andrew came around the corner into the family room and stopped dead in his tracks. Ellen was playing with her scrapbook and making a conscious effort to ignore her guest. Storm was standing up in the middle of the room, surrounded by a card house she had built around herself. The box containing all the playing cards Andrew and Basa had collected in their overseas trips lay open on the floor along with empty card packets, but it was the card house itself which caught Andrew's attention. It was circular, continuous, and wider at the base than the top. Storm was in the middle of it, placing layer upon layer with a precision of movement which startled him. The structure was waist high all round, and no doubt would have grown much higher. The girl turned round suddenly, and saw Andrew watching. She gave a startled yelp, tripped over her own feet and fell over amidst a rain of cards in every direction.

Seeing the wreck of her construction, or because her own feet had tripped her up again, the child curled herself up in a ball of dressing gown and began to cry. Ellen's huffiness evaporated instantly. She leapt to her feet, ran over to Storm, and threw her arms around the girl. After a second two arms came out of the dressing gown and wrapped themselves around Ellen, which had the effect of making her cry as well. Peter shook his head and sat down. Andrew, feeling as though the water was getting swiftly out of his depth, came over and knelt down beside them. He put his arm around his daughter, only to feel Storm's arm slip around his own back and tighten there.

"There's nothing to cry about," Andrew said comfortingly. "We can build another card house. Come on, there's really no need to cry."

Ellen turned big sorrowful eyes toward her father. "It's my fault, Daddy. I made her upset. She can't walk, and I made fun of her. That's why she started building cards."

"Did you teach her how to build cards?"

"Yes, but that was a while ago. She's good at it, isn't she?"

"Remarkably. Come on, Storm. Ellen's not cross with you. Oh, for goodness sake."

Storm had now thrown both her arms around Andrew, clinging to him tightly, just as a child would to a father. Andrew, feeling as though events had somehow taken charge of his reason, wrapped one arm gently around the girl and patted her back with his other hand. At this tender moment Basa strode into the room. She stared at the card strewn spectacle on the floor without saying a thing, but Peter knew that expression.

Taking out his mobile phone he walked over to his mother. "See Mum, she built that."

Basa took the phone from him and studied the picture silently. At the sound of Peter's voice Andrew extricated himself from the bundle of girls on the floor and stood up. He cast a pleading glance at his wife.

Peter explained, hoping to pour oil on troubled waters. "Ellen showed her how to build with a few cards and, well, this is what she did."

"Ellen showed her?" Basa said sharply. "Could she do it before?"

"I don't think so. Ellen got sick of it after a while and plugged herself into her iPod. She got sick of that too and tried to teach Storm to walk. That didn't go so well."

"Storm?" Who's Storm?" Basa said, her voice dripping displeasure.

Andrew came over and kissed his wife on the cheek. She didn't kiss him back. "Operation went well?" He smiled in an attempt to divert Basa into less stormy waters.

"Why is she still here?" Basa demanded. "Did you ring Brian?"

"Yes, of course I did. She's still here because nobody will claim her."

"Westmead hospital?"

"All present and correct. I kept annoying them until they wanted to murder me."

"Pathetic patient management!" Basa stormed, furiously. "She has to go. Andrew what's got into you?" She cast a quick glance at the rest of her family. "Have you all lost your reason? She's going."

Ellen pricked up her little ears at the sound of her mother's ultimatum. "Storm's here because we want her here," she said loudly. "She needs us. You can't send her away."

Basa knew that look of defiance in her daughter's face. How this sick girl came to have the name of Storm she didn't know, but she knew one was coming. Going over to Ellen she knelt down and spoke calmly and sternly. "Ellen, this girl belongs to somebody else. They're worried about her. If you were lost in someone else's house you would want to go home, wouldn't you?"

"Storm's not lost. She's meant to be here." Ellen stamped her foot.

"She's very sick. You want to make her better, don't you? She has to go to hospital so the doctors can find out what's wrong with—"

"There's nothing wrong with her!" Ellen shouted.

"Don't you raise your voice at me, young lady," Basa scolded. "That's all there is to it. I don't want to hear any more of this nonsense. This child is going today or I'll want to know why not."

Ellen's face dissolved into floods of tears. She ran out of the room leaving Andrew feeling more unsettled than he had in many a day. Storm was crying again for some reason, Peter quiet and thoughtful on his chair.

Basa glared from one face to another and shook her head angrily. "Has my entire family gone mad? I need a cup of tea."

She marched out of the room, a mixture of worry and anger on her face.

CHAPTER 3

Giving Storm back to her doting parents, carers, doctors or jailers proved to be an inexplicably difficult task, for the simple reason that nobody came forward to claim her. Andrew had gone through the same inquisitorial routine with every sort of hospital, private and public, sheltered workshop and psychiatric institution that he could think of. Brian had taken several photos of her for police files, so they could match her with a missing person.

It never happened.

The persons missing because of the storm were eventually all accounted for, some, tragically, when they found their bodies. Those who had been missing before the storm remained that way.

A whole week had passed since Storm arrived, and although Basa and Andrew had discussed it until they were sick of the subject, neither of them was the slightest bit closer to identifying her condition, let alone the cause of it. The lack of any diagnosis played on Basa's mind like the presence of a ticking bomb in the middle of her family, and each day she hounded Andrew to find some way of getting rid of the child. Her apprehension was daily exacerbated because every prediction she made concerning Storm's likely behaviour turned out to be wrong. The tumour would soon put her back in a coma, but her sleeping patterns began returning to exactly what would be expected from a teenage girl. The tumour was in a motor area of her brain, which accounted for her inability to walk properly, and soon they would see a marked deterioration in fine motor skills, then in gross motor. Storm's continuing disability was the cause of many tears, but on the other hand she continued to build card houses of great complexity, had progressed in bladder control until she was almost normal, and got very upset when she missed. She could now do a fair job with a spoon and fork at the table, and just yesterday made her own bed.

Brian Craig rang early Saturday morning. "The boss wants to see you pretty soon," he said, "this morning if you can. It's about the storm girl."

Andrew gritted his teeth. He had been expecting the summons, and was surprised Detective Inspector Ray Wright should have taken so long to make it. "Tell him I'll be there after ten," he sighed. "I've got patients before then."

It was a true statement, but Andrew wanted more time to think. Glancing into the kitchen he was just in time to see Basa grabbing her coffee and heading out to the Village for supplies. Thankfully he had been the one to pick up the phone.

True to his word, Andrew arrived at Ryde Police Station at ten fifteen and was shown into Wright's spartanly furnished office. A large wooden desk strewn with paper occupied a third of the room, and beige filing cabinets another third, leaving a narrow area of carpet with a black office chair which had seen better days. Wright motioned Andrew into it.

"Your brother tells me you still have that unidentified young woman staying with you." It was more a statement than a question, and Andrew saw no point in trying to fit an answer around it. He eyed Wright with a blank expression.

"I was wondering when you were going to report her existence to the Department of Social Services," Wright continued. "I assume as a doctor dealing with the public you already know it's mandatory."

Andrew cleared his throat. "I have no intention of reporting her to DSS. At present she's my patient, under my care, and I take full responsibility for her, like I do with every other patient."

Wright grunted. "Your patient, you say? What is she suffering from?"

"She has acquired intracranial injury," Andrew said slowly. "This has severely impaired her intellectual, linguistic and motor capacity. She has had multiple cranial surgeries, as you already know. I am not able to tell you why at this stage."

"Your prognosis?" Wright raised his eyebrows.

"There are signs of improvement, no doubt assisted by the environment and care our family is providing," Andrew answered, staring unblinking at Wright.

"And her memory, is that included in the improvement you speak of?" A tiny smile briefly lingered on Wright's face.

"No. Perhaps it will improve, I don't know."

"Of course you don't know," Wright said sharply, "because you haven't scheduled her for any advanced pathology or diagnosis. No Magnetic Resonance Imaging, not even a CAT scan. Why not? Because you don't have a name or a Medicare number to go with the face. As soon as you front up with her at any of those places DSS will know all about it. Why are you so reluctant to obey the law?"

Andrew took a deep breath. "DSS is understaffed and underfunded. What would they do with her? Put her in some sheltered facility with other intellectually disabled children, or worse. It would destroy the girl. No organisation could replace the healing care we are able to give her."

"You seem to have little faith in our social services," Wright remarked drily.

"I know what they can and can't do," Andrew said, trying to keep the rising panic out of his voice. "You've taken her picture, so you know she's an exceptionally pretty young woman. She's also completely naïve, which makes her incredibly vulnerable. She'd be sexually violated in no time. You might as well sell her to a brothel."

Wright gave a twisted smile. "Naïve and beautiful, eh? Seems to me you're putting your personal reputation at risk, as well as that of your family. How does your wife feel about this?"

It was the question Andrew had dreaded. He sighed heavily. "My wife is a very caring mother. She fears the girl's severe intellectual disability will place a detrimental burden on our children. Basa doesn't believe the girl will ever improve. We disagree as to the diagnosis and prognosis. The truth is our children would be very distressed if she was taken away."

"I'm ringing DSS," Wright said, picking up the phone. "You should take more notice of your wife, Doctor Craig."

Wright lifted the receiver. Andrew reached out suddenly and slammed his hand down on the hook.

"I beg you, don't," he pleaded. "Listen to me. The girl has had multiple cranial surgeries. You don't do that in some backyard abortion clinic. Surgery like that requires a top class operating theatre equipped with the latest gear. The surgical team would have to be highly skilled. Certainly the one who stitched her head up was. Beautiful work."

"Your point?" Wright growled, still holding the phone tightly in his hand.

"That sort of surgery costs at least a hundred thousand a pop when you add on the after care," Andrew continued. "Top class surgeons were involved. She would have been nursed in a neurological ward for weeks. Why is there no record? Who paid for it?"

"Would you mind removing your hand from my phone?" Wright said in a dangerously soft voice.

"Thank you," he continued. "Perhaps she's an orphan who inherited a fortune. She discovers she's got a tumour on the brain and books herself into hospital. They keep on trying to remove the thing. Finally the brain damage is so severe she loses her memory and goes walkabout."

"Of course," Andrew said cynically. "A beautiful teenage orphan, rolling in money, without a guardian or a single friend, pays a top class hospital and a specialist surgical team to remove her tumour via multiple operations – and there's no paper trail? Nobody reports her absence. She goes walkabout during a horrendous storm and apparently travels umpteen kilometres without public transport. Doesn't that strike you as ridiculous?"

A slow smile lingered on Wright's face. "Suppose you tell me your theory," he said.

"The girl never had a brain tumour of any sort," Andrew said forcefully. "She was operated on without her consent for some foul purpose. Criminal medical malpractice, that's what this is. Why hasn't anyone claimed her? Because they probably think she's dead – and if they ever find out she isn't, they'll make sure she is. Maybe they're searching for her right now. We're talking about skilled surgeons here, that's the magnitude of it. Sheltered workshops and the like are exactly where they would think of looking for her." He stared at Wright angrily. "Do you want her to fall back into their hands?" He slammed his fist down on the desk. "No, you don't care at all. Just make sure the paperwork is okay, isn't that what you people do?"

Wright scratched his chin in silence. He gave a sigh, pushed himself backwards in his chair and touched his fingers together. "Last week we arrested three men on child sex offences, two leaders of a local gang who were extorting cash out of pensioners, and a guy who knifed an innocent young man in a pub. Here I am on a Saturday, enjoying myself. You see, I just live to fill out paperwork."

He paused, watching the effect of this revelation on Andrew. He shut his eyes. "I'd already considered that possibility," he said. "Perhaps you could tell me how not reporting this to DSS would assist my investigation."

Andrew was somewhat taken aback. "My apologies," he muttered. "If you hand her over to DSS you've lost her. It won't be long before she's sexually abused, and buried in mountains of cover-up. They won't let you near her. The swine who did this to her will find her and silence her for good. Leave her with me and I promise you full access whenever you want it. I'll keep you informed. With me taking care of her your investigation goes full steam ahead. Give her to DSS and you're stymied at every turn."

Wright sighed and straightened his chair. "A true knight in shining armour," he said. "I take your point. Placing her in the system could imperil her life. I've got two teenage daughters of my own, Craig." He sighed. "Alright, I'll bend the law. But if there's just one complaint, if DSS learns about her existence in some other way I'll feed you to the cleaners and I'll let them take the girl. I want weekly reports. If I find you've concealed information I'll drag her to DSS myself, willing or no. Deal?"

"Deal." Andrew brushed his forehead with the back of his hand.

"You'd better make sure she doesn't wander off again," Wright continued, standing up. "I feel sorry for your wife."

Andrew stood himself. "So do I," he said, and marched out the door.

※ ※ ※

While Andrew was absent, Basa had gone shopping, and grudgingly bought some underwear for Storm. She entertained no notion that the girl was going to stay, but didn't like the way she wandered around in a dressing gown all day. Her childlike naiveté and trust meant she didn't pay much attention to covering up her body, and although Peter was the very model of a good son and treated her almost like a sister, he obviously wasn't blind to her beauty either.

Returning home she left the packet of underwear on Storm's bed and went to pick up the other clothes from a neighbour across the street who had a teenage daughter around Storm's build. "We're taking temporary care of a patient, a state ward," she lied with a fluidity which would have made Ellen proud. "I'll return these in a week when she's gone." *Even sooner*, she thought to herself.

Basa delivered the clothes to Storm's bedroom, only to find the girl stark naked except for a pair of undies on her head and a bra around her waist, her legs through the straps.

"Take them off," Basa said impatiently.

Storm flinched at the sound of Basa's voice and did precisely nothing.

Basa sighed, reached out and attempted to drag the bra free from Storm's legs. The girl clamped them together hard, and backed away across the bed. Basa made a grab for the undies and found her wrist restrained in a vice-like grip. There was fear in the girl's eyes now. The grip on her wrist slackened, and finally Storm dropped her hand. *She doesn't like being touched*, Basa thought to herself. With another sigh conveying her greatest reluctance, Basa shut the bedroom door and shed her clothes, making a neat pile at the end of the bed. She took her bra in her hand, lifted it so Storm could see how she was holding it, and put it on.

Storm took the bra off her legs and put it on exactly the same way.

Basa repeated the procedure with her undies, then selecting a top from the collection that Sharon's mum had given her, placed it on the bed. She picked up her own top and put it on, watching in quiet disbelief as the child did the same. A short time later Storm sat on the edge of the bed fully clothed, a satisfied smile on her face. Basa left the bedroom with a headache. The child was learning. How on earth was that possible?

Andrew arrived home shortly before lunch. Storm, fully clothed for the first time, bounced up from the lounge where she had been playing noughts and crosses with Peter, twisted her way over to him, and threw her arms around his neck.

Basa watched from the kitchen with obvious disapproval. Apparently the patient didn't mind being touched by her husband.

"You're wearing new clothes today," Andrew laughed, giving her a hug. "It's a great improvement over the dressing gown."

"It's a great improvement over the dressing gown," Storm laughed back.

Basa scowled and continued preparing lunch. Perhaps Andrew wasn't blind to Storm's beauty either. She tried to banish the thought from her mind. A carrot on the chopping board took the full brunt of her anger. Andrew returned from the lounge room a short time later.

"When is she going?" Basa snapped, shredding a lettuce with a good deal more vigour than strictly necessary.

"She's not," Andrew said uneasily. "I know there's things to talk about. We can do it after lunch."

Lunch was an unusually silent affair. Even Storm could sense an air of tension, and as a result managed to upset her drink and spill some of her salad on the floor. Ellen instantly sprang up to help clean up the mess, and Peter, as surreptitiously as possible, reached out under the table and squeezed Storm's hand. His parents rarely fought about anything, but something was clearly amiss.

After lunch Andrew and Basa disappeared into the surgery. Ellen suggested Peter take Storm outside to have a look at the garden, while she put the lunch plates in the dishwasher. As soon as her brother and his charge disappeared through the back door, Ellen put down the plate she was holding and slunk down the corridor towards the surgery door. There were doings afoot, and she wasn't about to let them catch her by surprise.

Inside the surgery you could have cut the air with a knife.

"Tell me why she's not going," Basa launched the attack. "Andrew, I'm very concerned about the way you're behaving towards the patient."

Andrew suppressed the defensive barb he was about to hurl in reply. "She's not going because Detective Inspector Ray Wright thinks it's better she stay in our care for a while."

He briefly related his conversation with the inspector that morning. The frown on Basa's face deepened.

"You're breaking the law," she snapped, "and what's more, you're damaging this family."

"I can see no damage," Andrew said defensively. "Our children care for Storm a great deal. Both of them would be devastated if she was sent away, and you know it."

"It's school holidays," Basa continued. "What happens when we're back in term time? How do you think they'll react when one of us has to end their career to look after her? Which is it to be, me or you? How do you think your patients will react when they learn we're hiding some disabled girl in our home, especially if they see her? Your reputation will be in the gutter. I had to lie to Sharon's mother when I borrowed the clothes. If she found out we were harbouring a demented child for no good reason I'd die of shame."

"I have more faith in my patients than you do, apparently," Andrew said. "Can't you take care of someone these days without everyone thinking you've got some foul ulterior motive?"

"How do you propose we help her?" Basa continued, ignoring Andrew's words. "She has no Medicare number. We can't perform an MRI or CAT scan by ourselves. All we've got is guesswork diagnosis, and we can't even agree on that. What happens when her condition deteriorates further and she needs to be hospitalised? As soon as we take her to any hospital, DSS will land on us like a ton of bricks anyway."

"Does she seem to be deteriorating?" Andrew spoke softly.

"Andrew, she's a high maintenance young woman with severe intellectual impairment, even if it doesn't get worse," Basa said, her voice heavy with exasperation.

"I know families with mentally disabled children, and the cost is enormous. Their other children suffer from neglect. You know this is true. Do you want the same thing to happen to Ellen and Peter? Once she's a ward of the state she can receive proper specialist treatment."

"Which they will pay for out of the sheer generosity of their empty bank accounts," Andrew said more sharply than he had intended. "She'll end up in some psychiatric institution. I don't have to tell you what will happen to her there." He groaned softly. "Basa, she's learning. Your diagnosis can't account for that because it's wrong, and your prognosis is wrong as a result."

"Basa snorted. "And yours is plainly ridiculous. Medical malpractice? Andrew, I know the hospital system, and what you propose simply can't happen. In any case, her surgery - whatever it was - has left her in a permanently impaired condition. Even if she doesn't deteriorate, she'll never improve."

"Then how do you account for the complete absence of a paper trail?"

"Of course there's a paper trail," Basa snapped impatiently, "in some private hospital, more likely. Every minute of theatre time is booked in advance. A surgical team has to be assembled, accounts created. The operations would have taken hours, and recovery time, weeks. She's been a long care patient. Of course there's a paper trail. The police simply haven't found it yet. Give it a week or so and they will, mark my words. Why can't you see this?"

Andrew sighed heavily.

"But what if there isn't a paper trail? Basa, we're all she's got. I know what you're saying about our family is right, but on the other hand I can't bring myself to throw her to the wolves. She's responding to love, Basa, can't you see that? You've seen the improvement with your own eyes. If we give her a few more months—"

"It's December," Basa snapped angrily. "Come the first of January she's going. I'll ring DSS myself. We have a good marriage, Andrew, but I'm not letting you play knight in shining armour at the expense of my family, and that's the end of it."

Ellen, hearing her mother's footsteps, removed her ear from the surgery door and sprang down the hall into the kitchen. Peter was just coming in from the backyard. With one finger on her lips she pushed him outside again.

"Where's Storm?" she whispered.

"Out in the garden playing with our neighbour's cat," Peter said. "She just loves Mr. Macavity. Perhaps we should get her a—"

"Storm's in trouble," Ellen interrupted. "Mum wants to kick her out."

"You've only just picked up on that, have you?" Peter answered gloomily.

"No, stupid. She's going to kick her out on the first of January. She said so. Peter, do something!"

Peter groaned. The thought of throwing Storm out of the house made him feel physically ill in the stomach. "She won't survive," he muttered. "People will do horrible things to her." He gave another groan. "What do you expect me to do?"

"Mum thinks she's always going to be a baby," Ellen answered, "but she's not, she's learning heaps of stuff. We have to make sure she learns heaps more, so Mum will see she's wrong."

"How do we do that?" Peter asked.

"You teach her how to walk. I'll teach her how to do stuff that will impress Mum," Ellen said in a conspiratorial whisper. "We start tomorrow."

Basa stormed out of the surgery, slamming the door after her. Turning straight across the hall she flew into the bathroom and shut the door.

Sitting down on the toilet she took a towel and wiped the tears away from her eyes. She felt wretched. She always felt wretched when she had argued with Andrew, whom she loved dearly, but this time was worse. Why couldn't the man see what lay down the road? Why did she feel so bad about Storm?

Each morning since that day, with Ellen's help, Storm had arrived at the breakfast table properly dressed. Ellen would steal into her bedroom well before breakfast, wake her up, choose her clothes for the day, and make sure she put them on properly. Storm, who liked her sleep, didn't always cooperate very helpfully. She would have stayed in her bed until around nine in the morning if Ellen had let her.

Peter quickly abandoned his attempts to teach Storm to walk. After only five minutes trying, Storm had fallen over heavily and burst into tears. When he had knelt down to comfort her, Storm had thrown her arms around his neck and sobbed into his shoulder until his shirt was soaked. That was the end of that. He decided to follow Ellen's example and teach Storm how to do helpful things around the house.

Basa was completely aware of what her children were doing and why. It didn't really surprise her. Somehow they must have got wind of the patient's immanent departure, probably from Ellen, who had a knack of hearing things she wasn't meant to. But what really astonished Basa was Storm's apparent ability to learn, and the pattern, speed, and permanency of her learning defied each and every explanation she could think of. Privately she knew her original theory of severe permanent intracranial damage was not in keeping with the mounting pile of daily evidence. While Storm showed no signs of deterioration, not one shred of her past had returned. Every new behaviour was one the children – and Andrew - had taught her.

The girl was still completely echolalic. She could say words but had no language, trotting out phrases from her ever increasing database at what she supposed was the appropriate time. She would come into the breakfast room and greet Basa with the words "Good morning my Beauty", which instantly ruined her day until she realised Storm was copying Andrew. Ellen thought it was incredibly funny, and managed to get poor Storm to say lots of things which would have got her into heaps and heaps of trouble under normal circumstances.

Peter would look daggers at Ellen each time she did. "We're trying to make her look good for Mum," he hissed into her ear, "not make her look stupid."

In nearly every respect Storm was like a teenage baby who could learn. There was no such thing, Basa kept telling herself, and yet this impossible person was living in their very own home. Basa was an excellent doctor, but try as she might she couldn't explain her own observations. Even Andrew's impossible scenario didn't fit. If some unscrupulous surgeon had interfered with the girl's brain sufficiently to produce the symptoms Storm had presented with the day she arrived, the damage would be permanent, had to be permanent. Why was she capable of learning?

No matter, she had to go.

Yet the family she was so zealous to protect from the burden of caring for Storm, were daily becoming more attached to her. This alarmed Basa greatly. Any gentle hint of Storm leaving and Ellen would fly into hysterics. It was school holidays, Basa told herself, and Ellen had time on her hands. Storm allowed Ellen to teach her and boss her around, was affectionate and sisterly towards her, and as a result a bond had formed which was getting stronger by the day. Short joys and sharp sorrows were all part of a child's life, and when Storm was taken away, Ellen would get over it. It would be hard going for a day or two, that's all.

Peter worried her even more. She expected her seventeen year old son to be instantly fascinated and soon bored by the patient. He would surely regard Storm's temporary residence in their home as simply unavoidable if inconvenient, and spend more than the usual amount of time out of the house with his mates like he always did on holidays. This predictable behaviour pattern had completely disappeared. Whenever she found him he would be watching Ellen and Storm as they played together. Always a loving brother since the day Ellen came so unexpectedly into the world, she could understand his vigilance. But when Ellen went out with her father to the shops or whatever, rather than go away and leave Storm alone, he would take his sister's absence as his opportunity to teach Storm something new himself. It was obvious that he loved doing it just as much as Storm loved learning whatever he patiently taught her.

But her main worry was Andrew. In medical matters they had always seen eye to eye, except where Storm was concerned. Rather than take Basa's side and investigate every possible way to get the girl back into appropriate care, he seemed more and more determined to leave her where she was, despite the many disagreeable discussions they had had on the subject.

Then there was the way Storm reacted towards him. Each day she treated him more like a father, and never like a doctor in whose house she just happened to be living. More surprisingly, he didn't seem to mind, which made Basa furious and all the more determined to get rid of the patient.

At the breakfast table each morning, she, Basa was the only one who never got a hug from Storm, and the only person who never gave her one. Perhaps the girl could sense the distance at which Basa held her. Well, at least she wasn't going to be the one distraught when the girl left. In the meantime she would continue to use her training to the patient's benefit, even if no one else thought so.

That very morning, Friday, she was following up a new lead. Speaking to one of her colleagues, she had learned that a well-published professor of neurosurgery, one Isaac Gilead, was doing research in Australia with the University of Sydney. Perhaps he would be interested in this patient's case. She rang the faculty and asked to speak to him. The Dean's secretary dashed her hopes.

"I'm sorry, Doctor Craig. Professor Gilead has returned recently to continue his research at the Massachusetts Institute of Technology. No, we are not at liberty to give you his email address, but if you wished to contact MIT directly I am sure they would be most helpful."

She thanked the secretary and rang off. A professor in Massachusetts was not going to be interested in any patient from Australia. She brought up the MIT website and searched for his name and research area under the Medical Faculty. Nothing. Perhaps the site hadn't been updated if he had just arrived. She might skim through his published work though, when she had time. Right now there were several patients in Royal North Shore who needed follow up visits, and she was due in theatre after that. Soon the girl's treatment would be someone else's problem. Christmas was only a few days away, and the first of January was approaching fast.

CHAPTER 4

Sydney, three years before the Storm

I f Basa Craig had made that phone call three years previously, she would have received a very interesting answer. Gilead was still Professor of Neurology at Sydney University, and that particular morning he was about to begin a project which had been close to his heart for many years.

The meeting room was hushed, every eye turned to the podium where Gilead stood. He gave a small bow and began.

"Greetings, my learned, illustrious colleagues, superbly qualified support staff, and highly competent technicians. Such a collection of expertise has seldom been assembled in the history of medical research. Rest assured, we are going to make history. None of you, with the exception of two of my learned colleagues, have been briefed concerning the project we will collectively be working on. We shall correct the omission shortly."

He waved his arm in the direction of the laboratory down the corridor.

"You have, however, seen the magnificent equipment placed at your disposal, and you already know your salaries are far in excess of those normally offered for medical research. These luxuries are not provided by Amity-Rand Genetics on a whim. They are provided in the expectation we will succeed. These are the expressions of their confidence in you, and we shall not let them down."

He balled his fist and brought it down on the table in front of him. "For the next however many years this project will be your life, and you will readily dedicate every ability you possess to its common goal. If you do not wish to have these demands placed upon you, I would ask you to leave now."

He picked up a document from the table and waved it at the assembled group. "Should you wish to leave, you must sign the legal document in front of you. It binds you never to reveal anything you have seen or heard within these walls. Then you will receive a substantial payout. There will be no other obligation placed upon you, no ostracism of any kind will be forthcoming from anyone who chooses to remain. I pause for a response. This is your last opportunity to say no."

Not a person moved.

"Very well," Gilead smiled, "now some more introductions. To my right – he indicated with his arm – from the Goethe-Universität, Professor of neurophysiology, Doctor Gerhardt Metzger. Seated next to him, Doctor Max Hargraves, surgeon and anaesthetist, and Doctor Jan Yanac, cellular biologist, both associated with ARG. To my left, Doctor David Ross, geneticist from Cambridge, England. Professor Lavro Festerhaus needs no introduction to those geneticists present. He will be working with Gerhardt and myself on the transgenic aspects of the project."

He pointed towards the rear of the conference room.

"At the back of the room, the gentleman with the long hair, is Doctor Kevin Lucknow. He is one of the world's leading experts on Functional Magnetic Resonance Imaging. Next to him, Doctor John Roberts with a similar standing in Positron Emission Tomography. He will be working with the gentleman on his right, Doctor William Yung, nuclear chemist who has joined us from NASA."

He lowered his arm and pointed to another group sitting closer to the front.

"On the other table to my left, Drs. Lowrey and Ammar are dieticians on indefinite loan from the Australian National Institute, and the three sitting next to them are Paul Krishna, Sally Brown and Pat Cornish, physiotherapists who have joined us after a somewhat taxing and rigorous selection process. I congratulate them."

He waved his arm at the others in the room.

"We would be totally unable to contemplate this project were it not for our superbly trained technical and nursing staff. I have already spent too long on names you are unlikely to remember, so I will not introduce them at this time. I'm sure before long you will be personally acquainted with them all."

A soft murmur of gratitude came from an uncertain number of throats. Introductions could wait. The important question was why were they here at all? Hargraves and Yanac were there at the company's direction, the others mostly because of the lucrative salaries and the promise of working with the world's best. But what was the project? Something clearly significant from the line-up of academics in the room.

As if he had read their minds Isaac Gilead continued, a smile creeping across his face. "Yes, I can see you are anxious to know the purpose behind your recruitment. If your patience allows, I would like to give a brief introduction to our work. ARG is a stem cell pioneer. They see in this new area of biology the answer to a great number of health issues which now beset the human race. Stem cell therapies are not new, as I am sure you are all aware. Bone marrow transplants have been used for a long time, and more recently, we have seen tissue and joint repair successfully carried out by the autologous harvesting of adult stem cells from blood or adipose tissue. Of course the body also initiates its own repair of regenerative organs, such as blood, skin and intestinal tissues using its own adult stem cells."

Gilead moved towards the whiteboard and picked up a marker from the tray. In large letters he wrote 'central nervous system' across the top.

"However," he continued, "there is one system in the human body which so far has eluded repair by stem cell therapies, the central nervous system. The effects of brain injury or disease are among the most distressing we can ever encounter. The slow, lingering loss of a loved one whose neurons are degenerating due to Parkinson's disease, dementia, multiple sclerosis, Alzheimer's, or the plethora of other diseases which attack cerebral neurons or myelin sheaths, is a terrible burden for any family. Disease aside, a sudden cranial injury can leave its victim a changed persona for a lifetime."

Gilead flung out his arms towards his captivated audience in animated excitement.

"Imagine, esteemed colleagues, if we could find a way to repair such damage. If we could say to these suffering people, 'don't worry, all it needs is some replacement memory, some functioning processing, some new neurons or astrocytes which we can provide.' That, esteemed colleagues, is the goal of this project."

You could have heard a pin drop. Thirty three pairs of eyes were riveted on Gilead. Some appeared astounded. Most of them stared in cynical disbelief.

David Ross was the first to speak. "Professor Gilead, I can hardly believe ARG would fund such an ambitious goal to the extent they obviously have done. The human brain is an organ of vast complexity, the cortex multilayered. Buried under the cortex are substructures, corpus callosum, hypothalamus, thalamus, hippocampus, just to mention a few. You cannot seriously be suggesting it is possible to regenerate the neural composition of these structures, let alone wire them back into the brain's existing circuitry."

A general murmur of agreement could be heard over the soft whisper of air flowing through the ceiling vents. Gilead smiled, it was the reaction he expected. Inside he was practically overcome with excitement. Outside his face wore a much more sedate expression, although the light in his eyes gave the lie to it.

"I do not propose we begin with all the structures my worthy colleague has enumerated," he said. "No, we shall begin with the frontal cortex alone. If we are successful, which I believe we will be, we shall move into other areas, the motor region of the frontal lobe, the motor sensory area of the parietal lobe, and so on. If we succeed we shall delve further into the vast complexity hidden underneath."

Jan Yanac stood to his feet, an incredulous expression on his face. What was the company's purpose in sending him here? To report progress, he had been told, yet now he detected another, to be the voice of reason amongst the dreamers, damn and blast their hides. No bioethics committee would sanction such work on a human cortex, and without one the project's goal was doomed to failure. There was a good deal more anger and cynicism in his voice than he intended as he spoke. "So what model will we be employing, Professor Gilead? Mouse? Monkey? Yet with these your goal is out of the question. Others are working in this field – have been doing so for years, and we know what little progress they have made."

"I take your point, Jan," Gilead replied, smiling. "What model do you feel necessary to reach our goal?"

"Obviously a human head," Yanac answered stiffly. "I don't suppose you have one of those handy."

"Actually I have," Gilead said softly.

CHAPTER 5

Sydney, year of the Storm

I t was exactly two days before Christmas when the volcano erupted, and from such an innocent beginning. Ellen had come to her mother to ask her what she should give Storm for a present. Basa had snapped, "nothing, she's only a patient, and we don't give presents to patients." Ellen had stamped her foot without further comment and plied her brother with the same question. This time there was a more positive response.

"Why not a box of paints?" Peter suggested. "She's good at making stuff, maybe she'll like painting. Tell you what, if you make a card for her I'll buy the paints and we'll call it our present to Storm. Would you like that?"

Ellen, her eyes expressing her thanks even better than her words, said she thought it was a great idea. She would design a cool card. Good to his word, Peter caught the bus to Pennant Hills and returned with a generous collection of paint tubes and several brushes, in time to assist in the family ritual of assembling and decorating their plastic Christmas tree. None of them attached any religious significance to this seasonal activity. It was purely a tradition which the family enjoyed.

That afternoon, Andrew fetched the tree from its large box in the garage. Basa helped to sort out the branches. Peter began stringing the lights, and Ellen clipped the branch hooks onto the stem. When they had reached the last branch, Andrew added the crown and Peter wound the last string of lights around it. Basa commenced the second phase of the ritual by taking a large Nativity Scene out of its box and placing it carefully on the low table under the window. It had been in her family for ages, and it was very precious to her. An exquisitely carved Mary and Joseph watched over the Baby in the manger. Shepherds and wise men in painted array gathered round on the outside, except now there were only two shepherds and one wise man left, more than enough to maintain the fairy-tale euphoria of love and belonging. Now that was done the tree decoration could follow.

Storm soon caught on to the rules of the game, transferring ornaments from their tissue wrapping to the tree with great care, and repeating almost anything anybody said which made them all laugh, because she mimicked their delight as well as their words. The task was finished well before tea time, and Peter turned on the lights. The family stood and applauded, then dispersed into various rooms to complete their own private preparations, leaving Storm staring at the tree in wonder. After a while she twisted her way over to the lounge and curled up on it, keeping a watchful eye on the tree at the other end of the room.

During the next hour or so a small pile of presents began to grow around it as each member of the family would make a furtive entrance carrying another brightly wrapped gift. Peter was the last to come bearing their gift for Storm with Ellen's handmade card. From her place curled up on the lounge at the other side of the room, the future recipient watched silently. The beauty of the tree and the enticingly wrapped packages under it held her fascination, and she wondered what it was all about. Tomorrow she would find out.

The pizzas Andrew had ordered arrived sometime later, and the family gathered around the breakfast room table where they shared every meal.

"It's hot," Andrew said, placing a slice of pizza on Storm's plate. "Eat it carefully. Use your fingers. It's okay."

56

Storm poked her topping, drew back and stuck the exploratory finger in her mouth with a squeal of protest. Ellen giggled. Basa frowned her disapproval at both of them.

Peter came to her defence. "We told her to use her fingers. She doesn't understand what 'hot' means."

"She does now," Basa snapped. "Peter eat up, please, and stop fussing with the patient."

Over the last two hours Basa had reflected on Storm's participation in their private family Christmas preparations and decided it was the last straw. What right had this sick stranger to share in such intimacy and enjoyment? None whatever. She felt violated, and now the violator was being served pizza by her own husband.

Storm waited until her slice was almost cold before eating it. By the time she had finished there were only a few slices left. Peter picked up one and placed it on her plate. "It's cold enough now Storm. Did you enjoy that?"

"Enjoy. Enjoy."

Andrew looked up sharply from his nearly empty plate. Storm had copied Peter, but only one word, not the whole speech.

"Would you like another slice, Storm?" he said, smiling. "Before Peter eats it all?"

"Another slice Storm, before Peter eats it all?" Storm copied the question in Andrew's voice.

Andrew picked up another slice and transferred it to Storm's plate as well. For just a second he thought she had understood the words she had spoken, but probably not. Perhaps she never will, he thought to himself. After dinner Ellen transferred their few utensils to the dishwasher. Peter collected the pizza boxes and put them in the yellow recycling bin. Basa set the breakfast table with a new white cloth and the family went to bed.

Tomorrow morning was Sunday and the family slept late. Andrew and Basa woke around half past eight, but rather than getting up, spent the next hour in bed with one another, and a very pleasant hour it had been. Now Basa wrapped her dressing gown around her body and headed out to the kitchen for a cup of tea.

The shriek could have been heard across the road.

Andrew dragged on his dressing gown and bounded out of the bedroom thinking Basa must have been electrocuted with the jug. Peter fell out of his bedroom door mumbling something about alien invasion. Ellen came out of hers like a trident missile launch, and together they raced into the breakfast room to see what on earth the matter was. A large area of floor was covered with torn wrapping paper. Christmas presents, devoid of their attractive disguises, lay scattered all over the place. There was obviously nothing left under the tree. Each gift was intact and untouched save for one which had been put to immediate use, and it was this which had precipitated the scream. Storm had found her paints, and was putting the finishing touches to a large artwork which she had created on the fresh white table cloth by applying paint with her fingers. The family surged forward.

Basa emerged from the kitchen with a wooden spoon in her hand. Pushing her family away from the artwork she grabbed one of Storm's arms, shook the paint tube out of her fingers and delivered several hard blows to the back of her hand in quick succession.

"Bad, bad, bad, hand!" Still holding her hand in a vice like grip, Basa turned to the girl, her eyes blazing, her voice loud and charged with rage. "Look at the mess you've made. One more and you're out – I don't care where you go."

Storm stared at her uncomprehending. Then with a scream of terror, snatched her hand from Basa's grip, turned and tried to get away.

Storm Dancing

She moved backwards, fell over her feet and landed heavily on the floor, got up again, tried to run, fell over and stayed on the floor, visibly shaking with fear.

Ellen, her face as black with fury as it is possible for an eight year old girl to be, ran over and snatched the wooden spoon from her mother's hand. "How dare you hit Storm! How is she to know you shouldn't draw on the table?"

Basa pushed her away. Her daughter exploded in rage. "I hate you, I HATE YOU!"

Andrew's voice boomed loudly. "Ellen, go to your room at once. Go to your room. Now!"

Her father hardly ever raised his voice towards her. She turned and shot him a wounded, betrayed expression designed to break his heart on the spot, and ran from the room crying loudly. Making the most of this distraction Peter, unnoticed, helped Storm to her feet. She clung to his arm with both hands, and he could feel her body shaking, her eyes wide with fear. Basa strode forward, arms poised to tear the cloth from the table. She suspected some of the paint had soaked through onto the polished wooden surface. Her face was still contorted with rage.

Once again Andrew spoke, not so loudly this time, but with a ring of authority which Basa had hardly ever heard him use. "Basa, look at the picture. Put the cloth down and look at the picture."

Most of the picture was enclosed within a blue rectangular border. Outside the border on the left was an insidious black shape with sharp, angular irregular jagged edges, criss-crossed furiously with finger nail ridges and smudges, black on black. Somehow its creator had instilled the very essence of fear and loathing into that shape, and staring at it Basa felt herself swallow rapidly as though something had caught in her throat. Within the blue rectangle was a picture of the room they were standing in, the kitchen table itself occupying central place. It was adorned by the usual breakfast items, milk jug, pile of toast on a plate and so on, sketched brilliantly with an economy of lines drawn simply with finger, nail and paint. Storm may have had no language, but her art

59

had done with powerful eloquence what her words could not. On the opposite side of the table were three figures, Ellen in sunny yellow, her smile drawn with great care and detail, her hair a swirl of yellow smudge. Next to her was Peter in green, immediately recognisable by the shape of his hair in brown. This time the artist had paid great attention to his eyes, and staring at them Basa felt a shiver down her spine. They were unmistakably Peter eyes, locked in an expression that somehow conveyed love and thoughtfulness so powerfully she could hardly look away. Behind these two figures was a man, his arms laid gently on each of his children's shoulders, powerful arms to which the artist had added bulging muscles that Basa knew he didn't possess. His face was shining with delight, the very image of protective power and love for the children next to him.

On the right hand side of the room Storm had drawn the kitchen. Only a stroke here and there, but there was no doubt as to what it was. In the kitchen was another figure in brown, her eyes small, her hair long, her lips compressed together in a thin grimace. With one hand she held a black frying pan, the other arm, drawn quite out of proportion, was pointing across the room directly at the menacing black shape which lay beyond it, one finger extending like a claw. Basa stared transfixed by the image, unable to drag her eyes away. This was not the work of some mentally deranged child. This creativity was off the scale, even for a teenager, and its horrible message burned its way into her heart. She turned her head to find the artist herself staring at her, standing with both hands on Peter's arm, steadying herself and still shaking.

Basa pointed to the figure of herself in the drawing. "You want me to go there. This is what it says, doesn't it?" She indicated the long extended arm, the black shape outside the blue rectangle.

"You want ME to go there." Storm shouted. The words were exactly the same, the message totally opposite. Storm wasn't finished. "You want ME to go there. DON'T YOU?"

The last two original words were a scream. Storm flung Peter's arm away and hurled herself towards the hall. She could hardly walk at the best of times, but the grief and terror in her heart made it much, much worse. Twice she fell over heavily, got up in obvious pain, and continued her headlong rush to leave the house, cannoning into the sides of the hall as she did so. The family in the breakfast room had turned into stone. Peter stood open mouthed and very white, Andrew, his face like thunder, Basa in shock. They heard the front door open, slam shut, and she was gone.

Peter found his voice at last. "She's not leaving like that," he shouted.

He raced down the corridor and flung open the door, but Storm hadn't gone very far. Catapulting out the doorway she had stumbled down the front steps and lay dazed on the path leading up to them. There was a long handled trowel sticking in the soil of the petunia bed. The fallen girl snatched it out of the earth with both hands. Raising it above her head, she brought it down again and again on her right foot.

"Bad, bad, bad!" She cried, flinching each time with the pain.

It was so very much the same act which Basa had carried out on her hand. Peter, standing in the doorway next to his father, heard the sharp intake of his mother's breath behind his right ear. There was blood all over Storm's right foot as the child prepared to give her left one a dose of the same punishment, but Basa had had quite enough. Pushing through Andrew and Peter she hurled herself down the steps and snatched the trowel from the child's hand, throwing it away across the lawn. Storm turned to her with terrified eyes. Finding herself unable to walk, she began to push herself away on her backside with her hands in a manner which greatly distressed her audience. Basa had dropped down onto her knees but made no attempt to come closer. By now Storm, who was not watching where she was going, had managed to push herself backwards right into the wall of the house itself. She turned her head to see what was blocking her path then back to face the woman who hated her, the woman who wanted to send her back into terrifying nameless darkness. She froze, staring.

There were tears in Basa's eyes.

"Storm, please stop," Basa pleaded gently. "I was wrong. I'm sorry I hit you. Please don't go away."

Peter had never seen his mother cry. Here she was, kneeling on the path, tears running down her cheeks, her arms outstretched towards the frightened girl. The sight made him feel suddenly cold. He felt his father's grip tighten around his shoulder.

"It's going to be all right, Peter," he whispered. "Leave them, watch. It's going to be all right."

Slowly Basa began to move towards the girl, speaking softly, her arms held out in front of her. "I don't hate you, Storm. I tried to do what was best, and I was wrong. You belong with us. My family loves you, Storm. We don't want you to go back into the darkness."

At the mention of the darkness the child tensed against the wall. A single sob came from her lips, and Basa, taking this as her cue, came forward slowly and wrapped her arms around Storm's shoulders, drawing her head against her, holding her, rocking her gently from side to side as she began to cry in earnest. As Peter watched, he saw Storm's own arms wrap around his mother and tighten there. He glanced up at his Father in time to see him wiping his face with the back of his hand. *Well this is something new*, he thought to himself. *It's Christmas and all the family are bawling their eyes out.* Little by little Storm's sobbing became quieter, then the occasional gulp, finally nothing at all. Basa never stopped holding her face gently against her breast, rubbing her back comfortingly and slowly.

Now she spoke quietly. "Andrew, would you and Peter come and help me lift Storm into the house? Her foot has been cut badly with the trowel. I think straight into her bedroom would be best."

Six willing arms lifted Storm off the grass and up to the front door. At that point Andrew took over because they couldn't fit through otherwise, and carried her down the corridor to her room, lowering her gently onto her bed. Basa ran to the surgery and returned with some swabs, antiseptic and bandage. Ellen appeared in the doorway. She instantly read the change in her mother's face, leapt onto the bed and wrapped herself around Storm in a silent eloquence which said to all the world "if she goes, I go with her." Peter and Andrew sat next to her while Basa cleaned up the wounds.

Storm Dancing

Andrew, stroking the girl's hair, spoke softly to her. "Storm, you must never try to hurt yourself like that again. You don't have bad feet. They are really nice feet, but they don't know how to walk properly yet. Promise me you will be nice to them?"

"Promise me." Storm said, softly.

"Do you understand me?" Andrew asked in a gentle voice.

Storm looked into Andrew's face with large eyes. "Yes," she said quietly, "I understand."

After a second's stunned astonishment the whole family buried her in one long, affectionate embrace.

They spent a long time on Storm's bed that morning, each member of the family telling her in their own way how much they didn't want her to leave. Even Peter had managed to mumble something about how he would be bored without her, and the adoring smile she gave him when she reached out and squeezed his arm in reply, was one he would never forget. He had wanted to say some other stuff about how he really enjoyed teaching her, and really enjoyed being around her, and really enjoyed the way she laughed, but he thought he might mess it up and be misunderstood.

Andrew went back to the kitchen and returned with a large plate of buttered toast which they ate on Storm's bed as well – something so totally verboten it became a treasured memory. Then, with Peter supporting Storm on his arm because her foot was sore, everyone went back into the breakfast room. Andrew had thoughtfully removed the picture from the table and placed it in the back veranda to dry. A quick wipe with a wet dishcloth had removed every trace of paint from the wood. Basa asked Storm if she could keep it because it was very, very good and very, very special, and Storm had said "yes". It seemed a bit of a waste to wrap all the presents up again, so they spent the rest of the morning giving each other their gifts which they retrieved from the floor. So passed the most unusual, and in truth the most unforgettable Christmas on Christmas Eve that the family would ever have.

Andrew finished saying "goodnight" to Ellen and Peter, checked that the house was secure, and headed off to bed. He opened the bedroom door to find Basa sitting on the edge of the bed, tears streaming down her face. He came and sat beside her.

"I'm sorry," Basa stammered before he could say anything. "I'm a disgrace, Andrew. My concern for our family – and my jealousy – blinded me to the truth. It still bothers me the way you warmed so quickly to the girl. Ellen and Peter think of her like a baby teenage sister. You never went with my diagnosis, even from the beginning. Why?"

Andrew smiled and wrapped his arm around Basa's waist. "Ellen discovered it first. She has an extraordinary gift of understanding, that one. Takes a child to know a child, I guess. Quick as a flash too, like her mother."

"So what did Ellen discover?" Basa asked tearfully.

"Storm could learn. Ellen treated her like a baby, and started to teach her. That's what startled me, because she shouldn't have been able to learn a thing. Since then she's learnt an enormous amount. There's even the beginnings of language now."

More tears ran down Basa's cheeks. "I could see it too, but I wouldn't allow myself to believe it, because I couldn't explain it," she said softly.

"I can't explain it either," Andrew said softly. "She knew nothing. Nothing of her past has ever come back, either. It's almost as if there's nothing left to come back. She's incredibly smart, gifted, yes, gifted. That picture she drew – it sent shivers down my spine." Andrew shook his head.

"It opened my eyes," Basa said. "You've been right all along. That black thing - it's some sort of medical malpractice, something really horrible, isn't it?"

"I've come to think so. Helps explain why nobody will claim her. Someone wants her to be dead. The girl can't express it, perhaps she doesn't even know what it was, but that black thing was real and she's terrified of it. Something was done to her, what and why I don't know, and it wasn't done by some crackpot backyard doctor either."

"And by a series of bizarre coincidences she comes here. How strange is that? Do you think there's a God, Andrew? Has all this come about just by chance?"

"I don't know, Basa, but I tell you this. Whether it was fate or chance or destiny or God that brought her here, she's in the right place, and if that black thing tries to take her away it'll reckon with me."

Basa turned her body around until she was facing her husband. "And me," she said softly.

※ ※ ※

The next morning Andrew managed to stall Ellen's pre-breakfast visit to Storm's bedroom so the girl would remain sleeping. He woke Peter, and brought the children into the lounge room where Basa was waiting.

"Your mother wants to say something," he said simply.

Basa blinked back a tear. "Your Mum wants to say sorry," she said softly, "and to thank you for the way you cared for Storm. Dad and I need to talk to you both. There's a department called—"

"The Department of Social Services," Ellen piped up innocently. "They're supposed to be told about Storm. If they ever learn she's here, they'll come and take her away and put her in a lunatic asylum where she'll die from abuse."

Andrew smiled at his daughter. "I suppose one ought not to ask how you came by this little gem of information?"

Ellen bounded over and landed in his lap. "I'm very observant," she smiled innocently, "like you told Mum I was."

Storm had come to stay.

CHAPTER 6

Cambridge, Massachusetts, year after the Storm

I t was the beginning of June, and the start of a new academic year. The Massachusetts Institute of Technology boasts a large and illustrious faculty of Medicine. The huge auditorium was packed with eager-eyed hopefuls who were to begin their study of Medicine the following year.

The dean of the faculty had given them a taste of the goodies which awaited them, huge workloads, sleep deprivation, and ultimately great reward. Now he was introducing their new visiting Professor of neurosurgery, Doctor Isaac Gilead, who would be lecturing them on cranial anatomy in the second semester of the year. The dean's introduction was long and flattering, and from its object's point of view, boring and pointless. Soon the students would get another taste of what they would expect in the coming years – from him. The Dean finished, and sat down.

Gilead rose to his feet and walked slowly towards the microphone. He paused, surveying the crowd before him. Just like the rest, he surmised, most unpromising. Perhaps one or two of them would distinguish themselves in the years ahead.

"May I congratulate you on your admission to one of the finest Medical Schools in the world," he began. "I am sure your presence here is an indication of your excellent academic ability and your potential to work hard for the accolades which are awarded to this faculty's best," He paused. "You think you have come here to become doctors, but this course is not about making doctors of you. It is about making mechanics. Mechanics skilled enough to repair the most complex, the most astounding machine on the planet, the human body. Within this skin covered miracle of evolution you will discover the finest mechanical engineering, the most complex chemical engineering, the most sophisticated electrical engineering, and a level of computer science which makes the very best of our technology seem primitive."

He turned to the student in the second row who was furiously typing on his laptop. "You, the lad with the laptop. What processor do you have in there?"

The lad replied enthusiastically. "It's an Intel i7 quad core processor running at three point two gigahertz, with sixteen gigabytes of memory and two hundred and fifty gigabytes of solid state drive, sir."

The Professor smiled at him. "So, you know your machine. You have good taste, lad. I hope all that computing power will be used to work on your course material and not play games with your friends. Myself, I find quite a modest machine is all that is necessary for typing out assignments and accessing your course notes on the internet. No matter. Your machine is capable of processing around one hundred and fifty thousand million instructions per second. Very fast. That is approaching the limit of our technology. Now perhaps you would care to guess how many instructions per second this slow old brain of ours, running entirely on chemical reactions, without a single strand of silicon or copper wire to its credit is capable of? That is not a rhetorical question. Some answers please."

The girl in the front row piped up. "About one hundred instructions per second. We can only process so few things at the same time."

"So, one hundred instructions per second," Gilead smiled at her. "You may have underestimated your brain a little, young woman." He paused, "perhaps not."

A soft ripple of laughter passed through the group. A young man at the back of the theatre ventured another try. "I think the human brain is probably better than the quad core. I mean, it has to do quite a lot of processing just to keep us alive, let alone do anything else. I estimate two hundred thousand MIPS – or million instructions per second."

"An improvement over the hundred," Gilead nodded his head. "I will take a third estimate from anyone who would care to give it."

Another young woman, this time from the other side of the theatre put up her hand. The Professor acknowledged her with a nod. "I believe God made the human brain, whereas we made the i7 processor, and so the brain must be much better. I'm going out on a bit of a limb here and say five hundred thousand MIPS."

A louder ripple of laughter rang through the room. Professor Gilead grimaced slightly and continued. "I am somewhat gratified that you ascribe so little to your god, young lady. Based on the number of neurons, the parallel processing, the rate at which a neural network can be established and read, the best estimate for the processing power of the human brain is around one hundred to one hundred and fifty *million* MIPS."

There was silence. Two hundred pairs of eyes stared at Gilead unbelieving. The Professor continued. "Inside that organ waving around on top of your neck, the one you poison with drugs and alcohol, is a multi-processor computer the like of which we have never built on the face of the Earth. It is deserving of the finest IT specialist, the most meticulous engineer. Mechanics, that is what you will be trained to be, the finest mechanics, for nothing less will do for repairing such a superb machine. Superb? I use too diminutive a word. Stupendous. Amazing."

His face became suddenly intense and serious. "But, and this is what I am going to get through your heads if it's the last thing I do – a machine, entirely governed by chemical law, electrical law, physical law at the very highest level."

He paused again and surveyed the room. "I applaud for her bravery the last young woman who spoke of her faith in some metaphysical being. Let me tell you now, all of you, that was the last metaphysical statement I will tolerate in my lectures. A mechanic who believes a car has a soul does pathetic repair work. Would you rather have your brakes fixed by prayer or a spanner in the hands of a competent mechanic?"

He paused, smiling to himself, "If any one of you is in the habit of praying for your Ford's mechanical problems, please let me know straight away. Some remedial medical attention may be called for."

A ripple of laughter rang through the lecture theatre. The good Professor smiled. "To attribute any, *any* function, or ability, or system of the human body to some metaphysical principle is tantamount to admitting you do not understand how it works, and therefore you cannot fix it when it breaks down. Good doctors, competent mechanics, know and understand the nature of the machine given into their care. Metaphysics is a retreat into ignorance, an excuse for your inability to do the job properly, professionally. It took hundreds of years for science to emerge from the religious ignorance of the dark ages, hundreds of years before people learned that if they wanted healing they should go to their doctor and not their parish priest. Those who remained in that prevalent superstition were the ones who died. Antibiotics and not prayer is the cure for infection."

He paused again, weighing the effect his words were having on his audience. "When you graduate – *if* you graduate from this course as a mechanic – a doctor – you will be a good doctor, a doctor who has moved past that age of ignorance with its metaphysical principles and its gods, and walked full knowing into the new age of science and reality. You will believe from the depths of your being that when you go to treat a patient, it is a case of one machine repairing another, one machine programmed with the skill set required to perform such humanitarian work."

He softened his tone a little, and bent close to the microphone. "I am aware there are those of you who have been brought up to believe otherwise. Your minds have been programmed – perhaps before birth - to accept such beliefs as truth. I know, I understand, and I will do everything in my power to persuade you of the mistake you are making, to reprogram your minds with objective truth so that you can reach your full potential. I have found such a transition is quite easily accomplished, and I am proud to say I have achieved this result in many students who went on to become fine doctors. Their parish priests were not so pleased." He smiled, "It remains for me to wish you an enjoyable and stimulating time at MIT".

Professor Isaac Gilead sat down in the midst of total silence. There were some other speakers but he paid no attention to them. He shut his eyes against the glare of the stage lighting, and wished he could get back to his laboratory. The report he had been expecting from the Bioethics Committee would be coming soon, and if favourable, would enable him to continue the research he had been doing. Right then and there he felt his phone buzz against his chest. That would be the call he had been waiting for. The Bursar was winding up his spiel concerning fees to the sounds of students packing away their belongings. The young man with the laptop had shut down and was transferring the machine to his briefcase. He stood up as the students began to leave and checked the message on his phone: 'Isaac, please see me at your earliest convenience' from Professor James Harper, Head, medical research and bioethics. Ten minutes later he was standing in front of the gentleman.

James pushed himself out of the chair behind his desk and came round to shake his friend's hand. "Bad news, Isaac. I'm sorry. They wouldn't pass it."

"I expected as much, but then there is always hope, isn't there?"

"One day. Don't give up, Isaac." James sat down again. "The research you propose is amazing, brilliant. No one has even thought of using stem cells for that purpose, and yet, if it worked... What a leap forward in medicine."

"Oh it will work, James," Gilead said with a grimace, "but that leap forward in healing will never be accredited to this faculty, not while the bioethics committee is infested with narrow minded irrationality." He sat down in the other chair. "What was their objection?"

"See for yourself." James turned to his desk and fetched the sheaf of paper he had been reading. He turned several pages to one which displayed a paragraph he had highlighted in yellow. "Here it is. I'm sorry, Isaac."

Gilead took the report from his hand and scanned the paragraph in question. After several seconds he threw the entire collection of paper into the waste bin on the floor.

"Offensive to the principles of human dignity?" he said bitterly. "How much dignity can you have when your lungs are inoperative and your kidneys and legs smashed to pulp? Yet that young man could have been part of the process, part of the great leap forward you mentioned. In a matter of hours no doubt his viable organs will be harvested and matched to recipients, and the remainder of his body burned to ash. And this is more dignified?"

"You don't have to convince me, Isaac," Harper said with feeling, "but not every person on the committee shares our worldview. There are two Christians on the board, as well as several others who indulge in what you call metaphysical irrationality."

"Who gain enormous satisfaction from being the effective little gatekeepers they are." Gilead took off his glasses and stuffed them angrily in his shirt pocket. "What if one of them ends up in a neurological ward as the result of a car accident? Will their earnest prayers save them then? No, but this research might have. They will end up an incapacitated moron. Such dignity, sitting in a wheelchair in their nursing home, their family suffering interminably as they wait for them to die."

"I know," James sighed. "Yet the research you have done in Australia has already been of enormous benefit…"

"Incomplete, incomplete," Gilead sighed heavily. "I am getting old, James. In ten years I may have lost the acuity I now possess. I feel my time slipping away at the hands of the curse, always the same curse. How religion has blighted the human race!"

With a nod of agreement James Harper turned to his desk. Gilead stood and strode through the door, his lips compressed together. *Allow irrational gatekeepers to get in the way and you kiss good-bye to any worthwhile research,* he thought silently. In the past he had found ways around them, but in this country it was more difficult. There were deep Christian roots in America which, like the smile on the Cheshire cat, still lurked around after the animal itself had been ridiculed out of existence, and made life difficult.

In Australia, with no such religious heritage, life was far easier for visionary scientists like himself. Muttering under his breath he walked up the four flights of stairs to cancel all the arrangements he had made.

CHAPTER 7

Before the Storm

Rachel Demarra waited for the curtain to lift for the second time and bowed low to the clapping audience, all fifty of them, forty nine if you discounted her sixteen year old daughter. She was glad the floodlights blinded her view, although she needed no sight to see the cynical stare of her daughter's eyes, the petulant twist of her lips, the bored slouch of her shoulders, her hands clutching yet another packet of chips which she enjoyed eating as loudly as possible whenever her mother was on stage.

The curtain finally lowered for the second time, never to rise again, which spared the cast the pretence of enjoyment and the audience the pretence of gratitude. It wasn't her fault, the play was a disaster. It would only run one more night, not the three weeks which its creator had promised, cursed with the one-eyed artistic soul which deceived him into believing his plays were the work of genius. She thought of the likely lines she would read in the morning paper.

> 'If Harry Donahue believes Demarra's perfect derriere appearing with monotonous regularity in nearly every scene somehow compensates for the absence of a comprehensible plot, he should think again.'

STORM DANCING

It wasn't really imagination, she had been the victim of similar reviews before. The human body was after all an art work, and she was an artiste extraordinaire. She mumbled good-bye to her co-star and told him to rinse his mouth out in the dressing room because she thought she was getting a cold. He nodded with weary understanding and walked off in the opposite direction. Now to duck around the back past the critics who wanted a piece of her arse and the men who wanted another look at it. Her daughter Felicity would be waiting near their car out the back, wanting to be taken to McDonalds for ice cream. Well, if she kept her mouth shut about the play she might get her wish.

She walked off the stage to where she had put her handbag, and pulling a long black scarf out of it, wrapped the garment around her head and let herself out of the building via the back fire escape door. True to prediction Felicity was leaning against the car, obviously chewing gum, something her mother had absolutely forbidden her to do. The girl was out of control.

"Bloody awful, wasn't it?" Chew, chew, chew.

"Obviously you can't appreciate the playwright's synergistic metaphor, the deep irony conveyed by the juxtaposition of desire and meaninglessness."

"Obviously you don't either. The audience enjoyed your bum." Chew.

"That's enough. Do you want ice cream or not?" Rachel opened the car door.

"Depends how much I have to suck up to get it."

"Get in the blasted car!"

They drove off towards McDonalds. Miss Demarra felt her delicate soul beyond the capacity to cope with the tirade of vitriolic complaint which would undoubtedly ensue if she was foolish enough to go anywhere else. She glanced across at her daughter, her podgy thighs wedged in the seat beside her, and reflected that this course of action, while in her own best interests, was certainly not in those of her overweight offspring.

Couldn't be helped, one's children should not be allowed to ruin one's own mental health. How was she expected to perform her best tomorrow night? Felicity's tantrums often ran into days of stage-worthy performance, long acidic speeches and passionate destruction of various valuable items around the house, deliberately orchestrated to bring her own mother to a point of nervous collapse in as short a time as possible. Ice cream and a sundae were definitely called for. In the stony silence which accompanied the journey, Miss Demarra found herself recalling the sequence of unfortunate events which had resulted in the overweight burden she had to bear. Her father was to blame, as he was for everything.

The senior partner in the law firm of Demarra, McLean and Standish, John Demarra was a wealthy man, lived in a luxury apartment at Kirribilli, drove a Mercedes to work and a wife around the bend at home. Helen Demarra was a gentle woman, and if she had married a gentle man she would have made him a comely wife, to use a somewhat archaic word. Under John's dictatorial, legalistic, moralising demands she was reduced to a painted slave, always preparing for the many important guests he would bring home to impress as part of the process of securing their custom. A beautiful wife is always an asset on those occasions, and Helen learned that her sanity depended on making each of them the brilliant social successes her husband demanded.

Rachel arrived somewhat unexpectedly on the scene when Helen was thirty eight. John had grunted his acceptance of the inevitable, and Helen had been delighted. From the first time she held the small child in her arms some deep protective mothering instinct was kindled in her heart, and she determined her little girl would have the best that money could buy. This sudden intransigence came as a surprise to her husband, but it didn't take a lawyer to see the way the land lay from that time on. A condition had been added to his wife's contract of subservience:

> 'The father of one Rachel Demarra will provide whatsoever and whensoever her mother determines to be the child's needs or desires. Should this condition fail to be fulfilled to her mother's satisfaction consequences would follow which the said John Demarra would regret'.

Storm Dancing

Rachel Demarra grew up in the shadow of his tacit agreement, spoiled, overindulged, and devoted to her mother.

Then the first unfortunate event occurred. Helen was diagnosed with cancer and died just before Rachel's twentieth birthday, leaving Rachel beginning her final year at the National Institute of Dramatic Art.

The second unfortunate event followed soon after the first. After what seemed to Rachel a totally inappropriate period of grieving, her father had taken up with a much younger woman from Indonesia, whose lack of grace and poise was more than made up for by her superb figure and, Rachel surmised, her skill in the bedroom. Rachel, who up to this point had had little to say to her father, told him in every way she could think of that the woman was a gold digger, a conniving bitch who was simply wheedling her way into his life for the career opportunities it afforded. The long and fiery discussions did nothing but drive her father further away from her. As a result she had no knowledge of his registry office nuptials until the night of her graduation performance at NIDA, when her father had introduced her to his bride. He couldn't have chosen a worse time if he had tried.

So began unfortunate event number three.

Rachel's performance on stage that night had been excellent, but nothing could compare it to the encore she gave in the car park afterwards. The scene took place beside her father's large white Mercedes. Mila Demarra stepped out of the vehicle. Father introduced his bride, and Rachel Demarra inquired politely of her new step mother the name of the Jakarta brothel she had worked for prior to emigrating. It wasn't perhaps in the best interest of happy family relations, but then neither was Mila's suggestion, delivered at unnecessarily high volume, that her step-daughter must have slept with every single one of her instructors, because everyone watching her final performance could see she couldn't act to save her life. By now a small but enthusiastic audience had formed around the two women, who by this stage were passionately screaming withering defamation at one another. Her father, slipping back into the comfortable darkness of the parked vehicle, had called the police, fearing the exchange of insults might escalate to violence. About five minutes later Rachel had made an undignified exit stage left in the arms of two policemen. The crowd applauded. Mila Demarra got back into the car and continued a long and vitriolic monologue all the way home. Rachel never spoke to her father again.

Three years later John Demarra died of a heart attack, which Rachel attributed to excessive sex deliberately employed by the gold digging bitch he married for the purpose of sending him into an early grave.

So began unfortunate event number four.

One of her father's partners in law called her into his office a month later to deliver some rather distressing news. Father had left everything to his new wife, with the caveat that 'Mila would take care of his daughter as she knew he would have liked to have done.' Whether this comment was an example of her father's sexually induced senility or naturally occurring cynicism was impossible to tell. Mila had taken care of her alright, and the allowance she had been receiving from her father disappeared before you could say 'revenge'.

A young actress, even a talented one, had few opportunities in Australia in those years, and it wasn't long before Rachel's finances – which had never been in a wonderful state – were reduced to the cost of a single good meal. Feeling deeply that poverty was not a condition she could endure for more than five minutes, Rachel decided the time had come for compromise, either that or she would be performing down at the local soup kitchen. She shuddered at the thought. She could have easily got a job in some restaurant as a waitress, but the thought of occupying her time in anything else but the stage sent revulsion cascading down her spine. No, it was the stage or nothing.

Roger Harman was a self-opinionated stud. Several of Rachel's fellow actresses had described him as candy coated misery, and confided their desire to see him publicly eviscerated for a number of different reasons with a common theme. Somehow he had managed to wheedle his way into a full time acting career with The Sydney Theatrical Society, whose excellence attracted large audiences to their regular performances at the Wharf Theatre. How he had managed this feat was a matter of speculation amongst several of his fellow graduates who had not. To throw herself into the arms of a man who couldn't be faithful to his own cat was not something Rachel wanted to do, but then her career as an artiste was at stake. Besides, he lived at number 13/13 Trafalgar Street, and Rachel, like her mother, was incredibly and irrationally superstitious.

After planning her seduction routine in some detail, she went to see him perform in one of his plays and flattered him all the way to the bedroom. She had pawned the diamond earrings her mother had given her to provide the capital necessary to create the illusion she was comfortably off, an essential element in her subterfuge. Roger would never think of inviting a financial burden into his home, and by the time he realised his mistake, Rachel had taken up residence and made herself an indispensable part of his recreational enjoyment. It was rare to find a woman who would give so liberally to his favourite pastime without any of the usual monogamous restrictions which women were so infuriatingly disposed to place on a man's pleasurable activities.

Then came unfortunate event number five.

After just four months Rachel became pregnant. To Roger, she thought, but some of those après performance parties had got a little out of hand, and she had come to consciousness in some strange places with even stranger company. Roger had been surprisingly helpful, but following a successful audition for a major role in a new Lucas film he had taken off for the states. After all, the show must go on.

Three months of nauseous misery preceded six months of bit parts in various productions and a few ads, hardly enough to keep up the rent on Roger's modest apartment. To give her credit, Rachel rejected the many offers she had from the sleaze merchants to make pornographic films. On stage, before a live audience, anything she did was art. Not so in front of the camera. Also to her credit was the way she cared for the small bundle which appeared two weeks prematurely in Camperdown hospital.

A single mum trying desperately to make a living on the stage with a newborn baby and without a reputation is not an easy task. Many producers rejected her without even taking her audition when she walked into the room with a pram. Nonetheless somehow she managed it, and despite the little Felicity Demarra saw of her mother over the first six years of her life, a strong bond developed between them. Somehow the child understood that being parked in child care, or parked with friends, or parked in various after school venues was a necessity rather than her mother's preference.

The last unfortunate event occurred on Felicity's fourteenth birthday.

Rachel had taken her to see her latest play. It was a disastrous mistake. Felicity had tried faithfully to follow the convoluted plot until the time her own mother had walked on stage wearing nothing but a petunia in her hair and simulated passionate sex with her co-star, much to the appreciation of the theatre audience who were waiting for that scene with eager expectation. Felicity found herself sinking lower and lower in her seat and wishing very much that the floor would swallow her whole and take her into some other dimension. After the performance her mother had searched the theatre high and low for her, and was about to call the police when one of the stage hands told her there was a girl crying in the toilet.

The journey home had been far from pleasant. Rachel tried to explain how on stage her body simply became a vehicle for the playwright to express his creative genius. She was an artiste whose skill communicated to the audience the essential conundrum of the human condition. This was true entertainment, appreciated by those with fine intellects and open minds. Remembering the wolf whistles at the sight of her mother's bare assets, the child had given a much more earthy description of the way the intellectually gifted, open minded audience had interpreted her mother's performance, and ended her long monologue with an impassioned "I've never been so embarrassed in my life" delivered at full volume.

Somehow, although Rachel had never understood why, Felicity's demeanour had changed since that night. In her innocent heart a seed of belligerent cynicism had been planted, and in the two years since that unfortunate event it had grown and borne fruit. To Rachel, art was pure and beyond contempt. To her daughter, the dirty minded playwright her mother performed for was nothing but an emperor without clothes, secure in his delusion of grandeur, naked for all the world to see. The audience hadn't come to be confronted with the conundrum of the human condition, whatever that was. They liked the shape of her mother's bum. How mortifyingly embarrassing.

They pulled into the car park at McDonalds. Felicity got out and strode into the building savouring the taste of comfort food. Her mother locked the car, watching her daughter's plump silhouette waddle towards the lighted building. She sighed deeply and followed. Life, for some strange reason had become hard of late.

She felt in her pocket for the stone her therapist had given her, a smooth black rock from somewhere on the Isle of Skye where faeries still wandered out of the mounds on dark moonless nights to dance their rituals on the moors. Ah, that was better. There was power in that stone. She felt its smooth surface between her fingers, turning it over and over in the palm of her hand. Peace seemed to flood her soul. Yes, there was power in that stone.

Power there might have been, but the stone was one her therapist in a flash of genius had picked up from a pot on the way to her office one morning. The story she had crafted around it for the benefit of her superstitious client had worked like the charm the stone was supposed to be.

Felicity took the double sundae she had ordered back to a table as far from the front entrance as possible. Rachel, after paying for their meal came and sat next to her, sipping her diet coke and trying to show by example that fatty foods made fat people.

"Why do you keep doing that rubbish for Dirty Harry?" Felicity complained, shovelling sundae into her face.

Dirty Harry was Felicity's name for Harry Donahue who wrote most of the plays her mother acted in.

"I've told you not to call him that," Rachel answered crossly. "I do them because... I like them."

"Liar. You do them because no one else will give you a gig. No wonder. His reputation is rubbing off on you. Why not do a play where you get to keep your clothes on for a change instead of prostituting yourself in front of a whole lot of slavering men?"

"Why are you so cynical about everything I do?"

"Because you just don't get it." Another mouthful of sundae went home.

"You better pray I do get gigs because there's no ice cream if I don't get paid."

"It makes me feel so good eating the wages of theatrical prostitution."

"Then try eating less. You're beginning to look like a whale."

A grunt was all Rachel received, and the fire in Felicity's eyes told her there would be no more conversation that evening. Still, there hadn't been a tantrum either. One had to count one's blessings, no matter how meagre they seemed. She sighed heavily, stood up and jingled her keys. "I'm going home. Coming?"

CHAPTER 8

Year after the Storm

It was now midway through January. Ellen had turned eleven going on sixteen, and in a couple of weeks Peter would begin his final year at Pennant Hills High. He had started studying in the mornings and now spent most of every second day in his bedroom with his textbooks. Peter wasn't just after a good pass in the Higher School Certificate, he was shooting for Medicine, and to reach his goal he had to come good with an almost perfect score in every subject. Storm would come quietly into his room and curl up on the bed watching him making notes and doing problems. She never interrupted, content just to be in his presence, as if she could sense the days coming when he wouldn't be there and wanted to make the most of her time with him. When Peter noticed her he would stop and talk about what he was doing, and whether she understood or not she loved to listen. When she wasn't with Peter she played happily with Ellen, who was wise enough to realise that the baby teenager who had come so abruptly into their lives was growing up faster than she was. It was strange, but it didn't matter.

Learning to live with a teenage baby had brought its unique share of problems. There had been funny moments, such as the time Storm had squirted half a bottle of dishwashing liquid into the dishwasher instead of the proper powder. She had watched in horror as foam spurted out from around the door just after she had started the motor, and continued to spread across the kitchen floor. Basa had come into the room to find her desperately trying to gather up armfuls of the stuff and throw it into the kitchen sink, looking very worried and scared. She had turned round at the sound of Basa's laughter, and the palpable relief and gratitude on Storm's face had made Basa feel quite ashamed. Andrew had come in and taken a picture. In fact an album of the 'Craigs' life with Storm' was steadily growing. Storm asleep on a chair with Ellen asleep in her lap, Storm gawking at pictures of herself on Peter's iPad, Storm building card houses, making patterns with cutlery on the table, curled up on Peter's bed, being taught by Andrew how to make a paper boat, painting on the easel which Andrew and Basa had bought her, learning to cook gingerbread men with Ellen, listening while Peter read her a story. Her art work was amazing. In a few weeks she had produced so many pictures the Craigs could have papered their house with them. The black shape, so prominent in the early ones was absent in many of her latest creations, and it fascinated Basa to see the way it gradually grew smaller in each subsequent painting, as her fear of rejection was replaced by the certainty of love.

Then there was the morning when Storm had refused to get out of bed. The family had assembled in their usual order in the breakfast room at five thirty. Andrew had an eight thirty patient which was rare, and as a result was in an unusual hurry. Ellen bounced around setting the table, Peter cooked the toast, Basa did duty in the kitchen. Storm did not appear, so Andrew sent Ellen to fetch her.

"She won't get up," Ellen announced loudly, returning from her unsuccessful mission.

"We'll see about that." Basa slid the last omelette off her pan and headed for the bedroom.

"She's crying." Ellen placed another fork.

Basa paused in her tracks and rearranged the stern expression on her face to one of gentle concern, then headed for the bedroom. True enough, Storm had curled herself into a tight little ball with her pillow over her head.

Basa sat down on the bed and began to rub her back. "Storm, can you tell me what's wrong?"

After a pause the girl's muffled voice came from under the pillow. "Bed wet."

"Never mind, Storm, accidents—"

The head under the pillow shook violently from side to side. Basa paused in thought. "You're not in any sort of trouble, sweetheart," she said gently. "Can I see what has happened? Please don't be worried."

One glance at what had happened sent Basa scurrying down the hall. She picked up the phone in the breakfast room and left a message with her secretary to reschedule her first appointment, told the rest of the family Storm was alright, and went back to the girl. Andrew was on to his second patient, and Peter in his room studying before she emerged again, steadying Storm with her arm. She piloted her to a chair and returned to the kitchen. A short time later she carried two plates of bacon and eggs to the table, placed one in front of Storm, gave her a hug and sat down next to her.

"I've only got a few patients to see today, Storm," she encouraged. "I'll be home early and then we can finish talking. Remember what I told you?"

The girl nodded and flung her arms around Basa because she didn't want her to go. Ellen came into the room and stared at them long enough for her uncanny perception to tell her strange happenings were afoot. She fixed both of them with an enquiring eye and voiced her concern. "What's wrong with Storm, Mum?"

"Nothing, Ellen. Storm has been a little upset. She'll be alright soon," Basa said consolingly.

Ellen eyed her mother with a disapproving you're-keeping-secrets expression, but her mother didn't elaborate. True to her word Basa came back early in the afternoon, collected a book from the surgery and a sheaf of drawing paper from the kitchen, and went to find Storm. She found her curled up silently in the family room. The two went back into her bedroom and stayed there for a long while, much to Ellen's rising annoyance. Peter arrived back home after a run to keep up his fitness, and went to take a shower. Basa asked Ellen if she would like to go to the shops for an outing, and the two of them left together.

Peter stepped out of the shower screen stark naked and found Storm staring at him. His first reaction was to snatch a towel from the rack, but the look in her eyes halted him. There was nothing resembling lust or excitement, even naughtiness, just thoughtful, needful curiosity.

"I'm different," Storm said.

"Yes, you are. You're a girl, I'm a boy."

"I'm different, see?"

The girl opened her dressing gown. Peter could feel sweat budding on his forehead, simply from dread should a member of the family happen to walk in to the bathroom at this tender moment. "Yes, you're a girl. Storm, please cover up. If anyone comes in I don't know what I'd do."

The girl wrapped her dressing gown back around herself. "I like different. You'll be cold."

"Yes, I'll wrap a towel around me and go to my bedroom. I think you had better go out first."

Storm handed him a towel from the rack and went out, leaving a very grateful Peter behind. She was innocence itself, but Peter reflected that his own innocence had very definite limits, and he was pretty close to them. After that one occasion Storm never again intruded into his privacy. She had the picture now, understood some of it, accepted what she didn't understand, and that was that, or at least for the time being. There was obviously more to learn, and that story would make enjoyable reading one day. Right now, Peter was a boy and she was a girl who loved him, just like she loved all of them.

86

STORM DANCING

For all her innocence and funny ways, or perhaps because of them, Storm was an easy child to love. The family had expected her to display the usual sort of behaviour exhibited by babies and small children when they are testing the sanity of their parents, but she never did. Deep within the heart of the girl was an overwhelming sense of gratitude towards the family who had taken her in and come to love her when they could have done otherwise, thrown her back into the blackness of wherever it was she had come from. These people were her life. To leave them was to die, and Storm knew it. Behind her every action lay this fear and this gratitude, and from the gratitude grew a love and warmth which embraced each one of them. Beyond their gates lay a foreign and fearful world, within them there was security, meaning and life.

Not that she was perfect by any means. Her first act of deliberate and gentle naughtiness was the appearance of small creatures on the walls. Andrew, vacuuming down the hall, spied a row of ants travelling along the skirting board. Returning with a cloth and a can of spray he discovered, upon bending down close to the floor, that each ant had been drawn with a pencil. Very lifelike they were, and doing exactly what ants would do if they had been there to do it.

Andrew found the obvious culprit, and the wide eyed innocence on her face almost made him laugh. "Storm, you mustn't draw on the walls. It's very naughty. None of our children are allowed to do that."

"Storm, you mustn't draw on the walls. It's very naughty," the girl replied, staring wide eyed into his face.

"You know what I'm saying, don't you?" Andrew tried to look cross and failed.

"You know what I'm saying, don't you?" An innocent smile accompanied the eyes.

Storm's echolalia was very much worse when Storm wanted it to be, and Andrew reflected as he stared into those big, brown, serious, innocently pleading eyes that perhaps all girls had some sort of built in defences which gave them instant power over a man. Ellen certainly did, but he doubted she had been the one to teach Storm the art which the girl was now practising with such skill on him.

A few days later Basa found a lady beetle sketched on the side of Storm's window, just where you would have expected one to be, and a grasshopper on the wall of her bedroom just near the bedside table. The small creatures were so realistic you had to take a second look to convince yourself they weren't real. Storm was the obvious culprit, but no one could ever catch her in the act. The line of ants slowly crawled down the hall to the front door, and other little animals appeared in unexpected places at unexpected times. Peter and Ellen enjoyed discovering them. Andrew pretended not to notice, and Basa wasn't willing to jeopardise Storm's steadily building trust. Besides, she had drawn the creatures perfectly. Just how had she managed to do that?

The one and only blight on this peaceful scene remained Storm's inability to walk properly. If she tried very hard and walked very slowly and didn't mind twisting around a few times on the way she could get to where she wanted. If she moved quickly she would nearly always trip over her own feet and fall. At first she had been content to spend much of the day curled up on someone's bed or the lounge in front of the television when Ellen played one of her videos. With her new found interest in art, and the need to move her easel to where there were new and exciting things to draw, the rate at which she bruised herself began to exceed the rate at which the bruises healed.

The crisis came to a head one Friday evening. Peter had been out at school all day followed by a prefect's debate, and Storm had missed him. Around nine o'clock she heard the front door open and his cheery voice call out "I'm home" down the length of the hall. Storm jumped up from the lounge in excitement, twisted around a couple of times and collided with the telephone table, landing on the floor surrounded by a lot of bits and pieces. Basa flew into the room, saw the ruins of the table that had come from her parent's home in Debrecen, and almost cried.

Storm saw the sadness on her face and burst into tears. "I'm sorry. I'm sorry. I'm sorry!"

She kept on repeating the phrase, over and over again, sobbing her heart out. She had upset Basa, and she hated herself for doing it. Suddenly she snatched her right leg in a ferocious grip with both of her hands, and began banging it up and down on the floor.

The sobbing became very loud after that. By now every member of the family was in the room, and Basa, much to her credit was kneeling beside the girl, trying to comfort her.

"It was an accident, Storm," Basa said gently. Come on, let me help you up. You can't sit on the floor all night."

"No." Storm shook her head tearfully. "Stay on floor. Can't walk, break things."

It took a good ten minutes of family persuasion before she was willing to try. Andrew collected the remains of the table and said with more hope than conviction that it was going to be an easy repair. Storm sat on the lounge and refused to move. The family finally went to bed. Ellen, who was first up on Saturday, came into the lounge room to find her in the same place, curled up asleep. She ran over and threw her arms around her neck. That woke her up.

"Did you stay here all night?" Ellen asked.

"All night," Storm said sadly. "Not moving again."

"But you'll have to. You can't live on the lounge."

"Can."

Storm turned round and buried her head in the armrest. Ellen ran to Peter's room and woke him up next. Peter, unlike Ellen, did not come to consciousness all that quickly. He sat up and stared at his sister, resisting the temptation to hurl several small items within easy reach in her direction. He shook his head to help regain his wits. "What... what's got into you?"

"Storm won't move," Ellen explained. "She's still on the lounge. If she pees on it Mum will be boiling mad."

"Oh, for goodness sake." Peter groaned, stumbled out of bed and went into the lounge room. True enough, Storm was still on the lounge. Her head was jammed against the armrest and her feet tucked in tight against her body, her back to the world. The whole configuration said silently "leave me alone."

Peter went over to her and patted her shoulder. "Come on Storm, you can't stay there forever."

He felt the girl's body shake with a single sob. What to do now? She seemed so helpless. He leant over, pressed his head into Storm's neck and put his arms round her, something he had never done to Ellen, even when she was very upset. "Come on, Storm," he repeated gently. "You have to be the bravest girl I know. You don't give up. You can't give up now."

It felt really good to hold her in his arms. He was being the man, the strong brother, taking care of her.

She turned her face towards him without making the slightest attempt to wiggle free. "Peter, I can't walk. One day I'll break something ... something... "

"Valuable."

"Break something ... valuable and your family won't want me anymore."

Peter listened astounded to the longest original speech Storm had ever uttered. He felt a prickling sensation in his eyes which he fought to control. "Storm, we need you. We'll always love you, even if you smash up the whole house. Just try not to, that's all."

The girl laughed, and the smile on her face gave Peter an intense feeling of satisfaction. He pulled her into a sitting position and sat beside her.

He felt her head nestle on his shoulder, her arm creep around his waist. "I die if I'm not with you. I'm broken, Peter. Can you fix me?"

STORM DANCING

"Oh, for goodness sake."

Her head snuggled into his neck, the arm tightened around him, like a child holding on to an older brother, seeking comfort and feeling safe. Feelings which had been slowly growing inside Peter since the first time he saw her, rose up and gave themselves a name. He was her protector, her strong man, the one she depended on for help and comfort, the brother she needed. He liked the idea. Ellen was different. She was his sister and he loved her, but she didn't need him like Storm needed him. Glancing down at the carpet he noticed her sketch pad, and reaching down, turned it over to reveal her latest creation. He caught his breath and struggled for control before he spoke. "When did you do this?"

"Do this at night. I couldn't sleep. Feel sad, draw sad."

"Oh, Storm." He put the drawing down on the lounge, turned round and wrapped the girl in his arms. There were no doubt, fitting words for the occasion, but for the life of him Peter couldn't find them.

Just then Andrew came into the room. He gazed in alarm at his son embracing Storm, then he noticed the drawing face up on the lounge. He came over and picked it up, stared at it, and walked back to the bedroom. Basa was sitting up on the bed expecting her cup of tea which was part of their enjoyable Saturday morning routine. The first part had gone beautifully, but by the appearance of Andrew's face the second part had run into trouble.

"She drew this." He dropped the pad on the bed.

Around the edges of the page Storm had drawn the family, each of them engaged in some physical activity. Andrew and Peter were running, Ellen was doing cartwheels, Basa was jogging with weights in her hands. Andrew was walking, Ellen was jumping, Peter was kicking a ball around. In the centre, surrounded by all this energetic activity was Storm, her hands flailing above her head, her feet twisted around each other in the act of falling over. Her face was towards the ground, and falling from her eyes were a rain of tears which had flowed into an enormous puddle around her feet, the poignant sorrow of her face reflecting up in it.

Basa caught her breath. "Where did you find this?"

"On the lounge. Apparently Storm hasn't moved all night. Peter found it first. I came in to find him with his arms around the girl, wondered about that, then I saw why. I wouldn't have known what to say either."

For a long time Basa was silent, staring at the drawing. She gave a small, sorrowful sigh. "I'm useless, Andrew. I'm emotionally involved. I keep thinking 'tumour' and ... I've become so fond of her, Andrew. She matters to me, and I don't know what to do anymore."

"I don't think it's tumour," Andrew said seriously, "but it's almost certainly intracranial damage of some sort. She seems to be able to learn everything else, why not learn to walk? She can't crawl, either, because I've seen her try. There's impairment on one side."

"Her right leg," Basa nodded. "She has sensation in it, and muscle control, but the muscle control is wrong. There's something amiss with the ambulatory circuit for that side. That's why she goes round. Her right leg turns her, and to stop falling over she has to accommodate the movement with her left leg. Her left leg provides whatever progress she makes. I've watched her."

"Concur with observations. What's to be done? We can't let her go on like this. Have you seen the bruising?"

"More than you have. I went into the bathroom after her shower and she's covered with them. It's only a matter of time before she breaks a leg or an arm and then where would we be?"

Andrew sighed. "In one hell of a mess. As soon as that girl needs medical attention that we can't provide, we're in very deep water. No name, no Medicare number. Brian still can't understand why we don't hand her in to DSS."

"I thought like that once." Basa reached out and gripped her husband's arm. "We're all she's got Andrew, I'm convinced of that, and if DSS ever took her, I think ... You don't want to know what I think."

"There are robotic therapies which may be able to train her neurologically," Andrew said thoughtfully. "They set up new patterns in another part of her brain which is working properly, but we don't have access to the equipment."

"Sally Owens does," Basa frowned, "but I'm not prepared to take her into our confidence. Everyone would know within a week and Storm would be taken away from us."

"We'll have to do it ourselves, I mean the whole family," Andrew said, nodding slowly. "But we'll need to explain to her what she has to do, and I don't think she's got enough language yet."

"Then that's where we start," Basa said. "We have to teach her. She's an incredible communicator. All she needs is words and sentence practice. Her echolalia is slowly disappearing."

"Agreed, but I think there's something else we can do to begin with. Stupid of me not to think of it before. I guess when so much strangeness is happening you don't think of the obvious."

Andrew went out that morning and around lunchtime walked into the lounge room with something behind his back. Storm hadn't moved from her place. Ellen had brought her breakfast, partly because she wanted to help, and partly because she wanted to eat breakfast in a forbidden area. She went off to visit her friend after that and Peter had returned to his study.

"Storm, I have a present for you." Andrew smiled towards the figure curled up on the lounge.

Storm sat up. Andrew took the crutches from behind his back and held them out to her. The girl looked completely blank.

Andrew laughed. "Stupid of me. This is what you do with them."

Slipping his arms into the cuffs and holding the hand grips, he swung his way around the room with Storm staring at him in open-mouthed and wide-eyed amazement. After making a quick circuit he came over to her and held out the crutches. Storm stood up, fastened her arms as she had seen Andrew do, and took off. Round and round the room she went, faster and faster, tears of joy streaming down her face with shrieks of laughter and delight. She flew over to Andrew, and throwing the crutches aside, jumped up and flung her arms around his neck.

"Thank you, thank you, Daddy, thank you."

Andrew hugged the girl around the waist, and planted a kiss on her neck. *Dad*, he thought, and really liked the sound of it. Peter, hearing all the shouting had come running into the room. He saw the crutches lying on the floor, his father holding Storm with her feet off the ground, the wild delight in her eyes over his shoulder, and thought how very much he loved his father. For the next few hours Storm travelled everywhere on those crutches, up and down the hallway – Basa got a huge hug when she came out of the surgery – out into the backyard, round to the front, up the side path to the back, into the back door, and so on, the joy on her face radiating like sunshine wherever she went. Basa came back from shopping with Ellen around tea time to find her on the lounge, sound asleep from exhaustion, her new crutches tucked in next to her.

That evening Andrew began the game. Teach Storm a new word so she could say it in an original sentence without echoing, and you could put a cross on the chart. He produced an A3 sheet of paper with a matrix of small squares printed on its surface. When all the squares were full, five hundred of them, he would take the whole family to Animal World out near Arcadia, one of their favourite places, and after that they would go boating at Berowra Waters. The next target, one thousand new words would mean a dinner cruise on Sydney Harbour.

Ellen immediately went over and crossed a box. "I taught her the most important word of all," she said. "I gave Storm her name."

"Its new words, Ellen," her Dad reminded her, "but I think you deserve that one."

"Storm," Storm put the word in a sentence, "that's me."

Storm Dancing

For some reason which was not apparently clear, all the family thought that was very funny.

Later on that evening Andrew knocked on the door of his son's bedroom, and hearing the "okay" from inside, walked in. He sat down on the bed, carefully framing his thoughts. "Peter, let me say no father could be more proud of his son in the way you've taken care of Storm. I just want you to be careful, that's all."

"Careful? How do you mean?" Peter put down his pen and turned towards his father, his brow knitted in a frown.

"Storm's a pretty girl, a very pretty girl. But she's not your average teenager, is she? I mean... this is coming out badly... I don't want you to get hurt, Peter. Be careful how you manage your heart when Storm's around."

"You mean don't get into bed with her, don't you?"

"No, that wasn't in my thinking. Just don't treat her as a normal teenage girl like you would, say, Jessica Stevens across the road."

"Jessica Stevens isn't normal, she goes round like a bitch on heat. List of boyfriends as long as—"

"You know what I mean, Peter."

"Dad, Storm's as innocent as the driven snow. Do you think for a second I'd trade on that and do something to her? Frighten her? Come on."

"No, I know you'd never hurt Storm." Andrew shook his head. "It's you I was thinking about. Don't imagine she can respond to you the way a girl of her age normally can. How do you feel about her?"

Peter thought for a while before answering.

"She needs me, Dad, she needs you, she needs each one of us. And what do I think of her? I think of her as part of this family, a young woman who one day will make us proud and thankful we took her in. It's like watching

95

someone wake up, like seeing all the joy of discovery and wonder that I saw as Ellen began to find the world around her. But it's even more with Storm because she's growing up quicker, and she's older. She's so vulnerable, so fragile, and yet there's just so much warmth and joy in there too, a child's joy. I don't want her to find out that the world's a dirty place which preys on people like her. I tell you this, Dad, if anyone hurt Storm I'd want to kill them. I guess that sums it up pretty much. I saw what you did for her today. You were fantastic. Did you hear her? She called you Dad. What do you think of that?"

"She did, didn't she?" A smile crept over Andrew's face. "I liked it, Peter. I'm very fond of Storm, don't get me wrong. I have no idea how this story will end though. Some stories end in tragedy, remember."

"If there's a God He should be able to see this one's worthy of a happy ending."

"I think so too. Goodnight, son. Don't study too late."

He gave his son a hug then went out of the room. *I've got a fine boy there*, he thought to himself, *a wonderful wife too. Not many women would have done what Basa has. I pray it's the right thing. If Storm is taken away there's going to be four broken hearts around here.* He dismissed the thought from his mind. Once he got thinking like that so many problems seemed to stand up in front of his eyes and clamour for attention. Even Annette thought it strange the way their 'cousin' had apparently come to stay, and some of the neighbours were bound to be asking questions and poking their noses in where they weren't welcome. No, this wasn't a good time to think about such things, especially as you were heading to bed.

He opened the door to find his wife stretched out on top of the covers and closed it rapidly behind him.

"Thought you were never coming," she said.

He didn't need another invitation.

CHAPTER 9

Cambridge, Massachusetts, year after the Storm

Isaac Gilead adjusted the position of the lapel microphone attached to his shirt and stared gloomily at the young man on the opposite side of the coffee table that someone had placed between the two armchairs for some reason. Perhaps in some debates it acted as a physical barrier in case verbal attack proved an insufficient medium for expression. The Chairman smiled benignly at both of them. The young man seemed nervous. Gilead hated these contrived debates with a vengeance. In the end they achieved nothing. However the debate went he was certain the young man would walk away with his irrational views strengthened, and there was equally no possibility he would change his mind either. The audience – who were they? Christians waiting to see another sacrificial lamb slaughtered in the web of his own words, atheists who wished to see another Christian impaled on the stake of their own irrational stupidity. No one benefited. No souls were saved or lost. Indeed such an accomplishment was a total impossibility, seeing as there were no souls in the first place. At least this was only University Television, not some National Network.

The chairman, taking his cue from the flashing light on camera one, began. "A big hello to all you folks out there. Each week Ideology Today brings you face to face with divergent opinions on contemporary world views. This is your chairman Cameron Delaney."

He paused, eyed the two men in the armchairs as if to ready them for battle. "Is there a god? Christians and many other beliefs say yes, Professor Isaac Gilead says no, a debate which has been going on through the centuries since the rise of early modern science in the enlightenment many years ago. Tonight, to put the Christian point of view we have the Reverend Gordon Shaw, university chaplain and pastor to the Evangelical Students Group on campus. To present the case for atheism we have Dr. Isaac Gilead, Professor of Neuroscience. Dr. Gilead also holds a Doctorate of Surgery, and is one of the world's leading authorities on neurological circuitry of the brain. Gentlemen it is an honour to have you both here tonight."

There was a pause while the girl on the production desk faded the recording of audience applause up then down.

The Chairman turned to Gilead. "Professor Gilead, why does a neuroscientist of your stature and dedication take time to champion the cause of the New Atheism? Why do you consider it so important?"

Gilead shuffled uncomfortably in his armchair. He scrutinised the young man opposite carefully. Yes, he was doing it again. The man was in need of medical attention.

He glanced at the chairman and began. "I would much rather you say I champion the cause of sanity, of rationality. Human beings are possessed of a neurological structure which enables them to reason to an extent and depth far greater than any of the other wonderful creatures on this planet. I am simply an advocate of its efficient use."

"You would see belief in a god as a misuse of this ability?" Delaney queried.

"Belief in a god is irrational," Gilead responded with a sigh. "It makes no sense. If that was all I would not object so much, but this particular form of irrationality is destructive. When you say belief in god you have to ask which one? There are so many, and they contradict one another. If they are all descriptions of the same god it must suffer from unprecedented cosmic schizophrenia, a contradiction in being as well as personality. It is part of everything, it is personal, it is loving, it is merciless, it is indifferent,

98

it is concerned, I could go on. That's not the tragedy. The irrational servitude which human beings offer to whatever version of this god they hold has resulted in more bloodshed, violence and depravity than any other single cause throughout the gamut of human history. We are all part of the same human race. United in brotherhood, accepting what we are, we could achieve great things. But instead we fight, we slaughter, we defend our beliefs in the god of our choosing, none of which are either rational or open to verification."

Gilead paused, folded his hand back on his lap and politely waited for a reply from the other side of the coffee table. Reverend Shaw wasn't slow in providing it.

"There are many different beliefs I grant you, but only one correct belief—"

"My point exactly," Gilead interrupted. "Now you are going to tell me that your particular belief, for which you can offer no rational argument, is right and all the others are wrong. Wars have begun on similar claims. I trust one is not going to begin tonight."

"I have no intention of going to war with Professor Gilead," the Reverend Shaw said hastily, "but I must challenge his last statement. Christian belief is not based on irrationality but on the historical resurrection of the God – Man Jesus Christ from the dead. The birth, death, and resurrection of Jesus were prophesied thousands of years before they took place. We have copies of these documents dated at least one hundred years before the event itself took place. Let me ask the good Professor a question. If Jesus Christ did rise from the dead subsequent to his crucifixion, would he take seriously the claims to deity Jesus made about himself?"

Professor Gilead smiled at the young man sitting opposite. He seemed a decent sort of person, not at all like some of the vitriolic damn-you-in-hell types he had had the misfortune to debate with before.

He answered as gently as he could.

"I would, I would take them most seriously. I feel there are several other questions I would like to ask this resurrectee as well – concerning the process of regeneration of dead tissue – but I suppose if you're God you can do anything, even make matter out of nothing, produce energy out of the void, make white out of black."

"Then has Professor Gilead ever considered the incontrovertible historical evidence concerning the resurrection of Jesus?" The Reverend Shaw continued without raising his voice. "At what point did he feel the evidence was unconvincing?"

Professor Gilead reached inside his coat pocket and produced a small volume. He placed the book on his knee and smoothed the paper cover with his left hand. "Reverend Shaw, I have on my knee a history book. In this book the author tells me the atrocities against the Jews – like me – committed in places such as Auschwitz, never happened. The whole atrocity scenario was apparently nothing more than Jewish propaganda put forward to inflame hatred of the Nazis after the war. I would ask him if he subscribes to this view."

"Of course not." Reverend Shaw answered indignantly.

"Indeed I am glad to hear it," Gilead continued, "because my own grandfather and grandmother suffered horribly in that very place. I will not darken the evening by furthering a description of the depravity they endured. My point is this. How many years have run their course since those deplorable days? Sixty. Within sixty years we have history books which fundamentally disagree with one another on a matter of unprecedented genocide. History is subjective, my friend, guided far more by the political persuasion and financial interests of those who penned the documents than objective truth. Two thousand years of self-interested creativity must render any historical account of that age an unreliable fiction, unless Reverend Shaw is going to involve the mysterious hand of God again. If he does it is an unanswerable argument, unable to be proved or disproved."

"In that case the good Professor will disregard Julius Caesar as a figure of history," Shaw countered.

"The good Professor doesn't really care." Gilead smiled at his opponent and replaced the book in his coat pocket. "I know by this time the ancient historians in the audience will be throwing up their hands in horror. May I plead only that I am a humble man who likes to see the things he believes in, see them by whatever means, measure them, then use such measurements to benefit the human race."

"Surely you don't contend that reality must be measured in order to be reality," Reverend Shaw sounded incredulous.

"If it can't be measured, then what is the point of the discussion?" Gilead replied. "You say something is there, I say it isn't, and we waste a lot of our lives arguing an unprovable point. In the end, seeing as there is no measurement that either of us can make which proves or disproves the existence of this something, what possible benefit can there be to our discussion? What practical difference can it make to either of our lives?"

"I would contest that as an atheist you do not have the ability to see what every Christian knows by faith." There was an edge to the Reverend Shaw's voice, his hands gripped the armrests on his chair.

"Ah," Gilead smiled, "but I do have powers of observation which may be of greater benefit. For example, I have observed that when you look at me or our excellent chairman you turn your head a little too far to the left. Are you having trouble with the vision in your left eye?"

"I beg your pardon?"

The question was clearly one the Reverend Shaw did not expect.

"Your left eye," Gilead repeated gently. "Can you see out of it properly?"

"Err, no, my vision is a little blurred," Shaw blustered. "Perhaps I'm tired."

"And has it been that way for very long?"

At this point the chairman decided it was time to refocus the debate. He held up his hands towards his guests. "Gentlemen, I believe now is not the time to be speaking of personal matters such as eyesight. I am sure Professor Gilead has more to say on the topic we were discussing."

Gilead turned towards him with a smile. "On the contrary, Mr. Delaney, the Reverend Shaw's eyesight is entirely relevant. The man is suffering from a serious condition in his left eye, possibly glaucoma. If this is the case and it remains untreated for long he will go blind in that eye."

The Reverend Shaw stared at him as though he had just lost grip on the reality he had been talking about. "What?"

"I would ask the Reverend Shaw if the god he believes in is beneficent or indifferent to the health of his left eye," Gilead said in the same quiet voice. "Well?"

"God tells us in His Word that He knows every hair on my head. Of course He's not indifferent." Reverend Shaw began to sound defensive.

"And would you also concur your god answers prayer?"

"I would. I fail to see—"

"Then," Gilead interrupted, "would you please pray to your god and ask him to heal your eye immediately."

"I... I don't know if God wants to heal my eye immediately, I mean He hasn't told me... Perhaps in a day or two..." Small beads of sweat had formed on the Reverend Shaw's forehead.

"Very well. Pray that your god would heal your eye at his convenience, and then promise me and the audience who are listening to this program that you will never go near a doctor or an optometrist to seek a medical opinion."

"I...I would be foolish not to ask for appropriate medical help. God works through doctors and optometrists."

"But is he able to heal your eye directly," Gilead persisted, "or does he need the optometrists and doctors which all the unbelievers like me need? In which case believing in your god makes, as I have said, no difference."

"He can heal me directly - if He wants to," Shaw countered.

"Then ask him. Or do you doubt he may not be as beneficent as you like to believe?"

"Sometimes God does not work the way we would like Him to," Shaw said defensively.

"You mean the way he allowed six million Jews to perish in the gas chambers?" Gilead leaned forward in his chair. "Are you going to tell me none of them prayed for deliverance? No wonder you have doubts about his willingness to heal your eye when he turned a blind one to genocide. Such a god is surely worthy of reprimand, wouldn't you say?"

"I... don't know why... I'm not God... "

The Reverend Shaw was showing signs of stress.

Gilead frowned and stood up, detaching the microphone from his shirt. "This debate is causing the Reverend Shaw some stress, which is probably raising his blood pressure and increasing the risk to his eye. I will not continue under these circumstances. I leave you to wind up with our audience, Mr. Delaney. Reverend Shaw, will you go and see a qualified optometrist as soon as possible? Even one who doesn't believe in god?"

"I... yes, I will, and thank you." Shaw ripped the microphone from his coat and stood up.

"My pleasure," Gilead said. "Now if you will both excuse me I have other and perhaps more valuable work to do."

The Reverend Shaw walked out of the studio with the appearance of a man who has just been hit on the head with a blunt object. Delaney wound up the show twenty minutes early with a five minute palaver guaranteed to make his audience change channel, and in the middle of it the producer cut to a music video in order to keep them watching.

Chapter 10

Before the Storm

Rachel Demarra entered her apartment in Forest Lodge and slammed the door. The sound caused her daughter Felicity to push 'pause' on the remote, uncurl herself from the sofa and turn round to face the bedraggled mess coming down the hall.

"You're soaked," she said. "Is it raining, or were you performing some deep incomprehensible metaphor with a fire hose on stage?"

"It's teeming," Rachel snapped, "can't you hear it over the drivel you've been glued to all night?"

"I can now. Where's your umbrella?"

"You tell me where it is. In your bedroom under piles of rubbish I expect."

"So the play went well then." There was a cynical smile on Felicity's face.

"Harry's destroying his genius with booze." Rachel shucked off her sodden shoes.

"'Bout bloody time something put an end to it," Felicity returned. "Here's to the purifying effect of whiskey."

Rachel groaned. "You have no artistic soul."

"Thank goodness." Felicity put down the remote. "Why don't you get a job at McDonalds? I'd be a good customer."

"I'd rather die," Rachel answered passionately.

"There's an enormous demand for dead bodies in plays," Felicity smiled sweetly. "Wheel them in, wheel them off, stick them back in formaldehyde. I could be your manager, all you'd need is dusting off before opening night."

"You're giving your mother a terrible headache – after all I've been through tonight," Rachel complained. "I pour my heart into Donahue's script and all I get is derision – at home and the theatre. They had to take Jack Matthews to hospital after act three. Someone threw a bong at him."

Felicity laughed outright. "No doubt a complex metaphorical message from the audience."

"The play had to stop," Rachel continued. "Police were called. Quite a lot of the audience disappeared before they arrived. Seems there was some drug dealing going on in the back of the theatre, and one of them must have been a bit high."

"And that was the end?" Felicity reached for the remote again.

"No, the play went on without him."

"Anybody notice the difference?"

"I'm going to bed," Rachel snapped. "Enjoy the elitist trash you're watching."

"Goodnight." Felicity pushed 'play'.

The phone rang. It was one of those old fashioned phones attached to the wall in the hallway, and the sound of it ringing would have woken the dead, if they had been anywhere around to hear it. Felicity pushed 'pause', Rachel groaned again, walked over and picked up the receiver. It was Roger Harman calling from the Gold Coast.

"Roger!" Rachel screamed excitedly. "You're back in Oz. What are you... Oh. Wonderful... they need what? You mentioned me? You did? Roger! You're a saint. Love you darling. You do? Okay, when? Yes of course I'll be there. Can't wait. 'Bye.'"

By this time Felicity was all ears. Her biological father wasn't dead after all. Damnable shame, and worse still, he was somewhere on the same land mass as the unfortunate offspring of his promiscuity. Catastrophe. Her mother was beaming with desire, putting her eggs in jeopardy again. It had happened once, it could happen again, and then she would have a sibling to contend with. Drastic action had to be taken, but what? She glanced around the room for something valuable to destroy while she staged the tantrum of her life, and found it singularly absent of suitable targets. There was always the television, but if she destroyed that she knew her mother wouldn't replace it, and she would be the loser, big time. All the vases which Rachel had brought from her home had already made the supreme sacrifice, along with some expensive and irreplaceable crystal from the same source.

She picked up the remote – a girl has to compromise – and hurled it against the wall. "Don't you dare think of sniffing around that pile of promiscuous slime. Pick up the phone and tell him to pee off. Better still, let me call him. Let his ever-loving daughter tell her daddy what he can do with himself. Better cover your ears, it won't be pretty."

Rachel flinched at the sound of the remote disintegrating on the wall, then turned and fixed her daughter with a steely eye of determination. Felicity didn't like that steely eye, it meant her mother had made up her mind and was prepared to batten down hatches and weather the storm. Damn and blast the man.

"Roger has managed to get me an audition for a major part in a Universal picture," Rachel attempted explanation. "Can't you see what this means? No more doing rubbish for Donahue. We would have money to burn, people would turn their heads – 'there goes Rachel Demarra.' I would be famous."

"For showing your bum to the world."

"Felicity," Rachel warned, "I don't care if you like it or if you don't like it. I don't care if you come or you stay here all your life, but I'm going to see Roger, and I'm going to that audition. Make up your mind, and do it quickly."

Felicity sized her mother up. Yes, there was no stopping her once the lure of fame and fortune beckoned. A trip to the Gold Coast would be a welcome relief from the interminable boredom of Forest Lodge High, juvenile drug distribution centre for the inner West.

She arranged her face into the appropriate expression of disgust. "As long as I don't have to see him, hear him, speak to him or touch him. One winkle of his face and I'll scream abuse."

"Deal," her mother snapped. "I wouldn't want him to see you looking like a beached whale. You could be so attractive if you only slimmed down to half your size."

"It keeps my stomach happy and the sleazebags off. When do we go? Are we flying up there?"

"Day after tomorrow, and we'll go by train. No point in spending all that money. I'll have to go out and buy something suitable to wear."

"I need another swimming costume," Felicity interrupted. "You'd be surprised how sexy I look in one that's three sizes too small."

"Alright," Rachel groaned.

"Careful you don't spend too much accessorising or we'll be walking to the Gold Coast. I take it we're staying in some nice hotel?"

"Roger has asked us to stay with him in—"

"I'll scream abuse. Want a demonstration?"

"I'll get you a separate room on another floor," Rachel shuddered at the thought. "You think I want my daughter to ruin the only chance I get?"

"To roll over for the slime? You were better on stage."

"That's quite enough, Felicity," Rachel's voice quivered with emotion. "My love life is my own business."

"I heard of a girl who fed her baby sister to the crocodiles at Taronga Zoo."

"Spare me!" Her mother threw up her arms in horror and left the room. Felicity picked up the remains of the remote and attempted reassembly. The circuit board wasn't damaged, and in a few minutes she was back watching her elitist trash. The thought of accidentally running into Roger Harman needed diluting before she was ready to go to bed. On the screen the heroine had just successfully poisoned her faithless lover, and Felicity began to wonder just where you would go to get a syringe of the same stuff, and if it was expensive. Two hours later she switched off the player and went to bed.

Rachel had left the house before she got up and arrived back around afternoon tea time, laden with designer labelled bags and two airline tickets. Apparently the thought of all that train travel had made her change her mind. Perhaps it was simply the desire to spend tomorrow night with Roger rather than bumping along in an uncomfortable all night train and arriving far from her alluring best. This was the first time Felicity had travelled by plane, and the thought of rubbing shoulders with clouds rather excited her.

They left for the airport the next morning. There was a short bus ride to Central Station, a short train ride to the Domestic Terminal, and a disappointingly short flight to the Gold Coast. Felicity sat glued to the window as the magnificent Australian coastline spread out underneath her, and thought how very much she would love to be a pilot and fly over scenery like this day after day. She was smart enough. Without making any effort at all she had topped her year in Maths, English and Art. Several of her pictures were now in the foyer for visiting parents to admire.

Her enjoyment had slowly morphed into an uneasy vigilance as the taxi took them from the airport to the hotel where Harman was staying. Rachel bounded out of the taxi and stared around as though she expected Roger to be in the foyer panting with anticipation. Felicity stepped out of the taxi like a plump gazelle sniffing the air for hyenas. Rachel collected the key to her daughter's room and the child took off like the same gazelle, who whilst not actually spotting any hyenas, expected them to turn up any second and wasn't waiting around to be lunch.

Rachel enquired as to the whereabouts of Mr. Roger Harman and was told he was out all day with appointments, but had instructed the desk to give her a key to his room and suggest she make herself comfortable. She knew how to interpret that message. On arriving in his suite she found an envelope addressed to her with details of the audition, and a couple of pages of script. After a shower and the selection of suitably seductive attire, she lay down on the bed and began to learn her part. By the time Roger arrived for the anticipated evening's pleasures she had managed to memorise the lot.

It was nine pm before the couple, suitably tired from the strenuous exercise, arrived in the dining room. Felicity had been and gone long since, anticipating quite correctly that her mother and the slime would not arrive until much later. She had stuffed herself with a good deal more food than necessary and gone back to her room to watch cable television. There were some shows on cable they couldn't watch at home.

STORM DANCING

After a refreshing night's sleep Felicity woke early, went to the window, and saw the tree lined pool several stories below. The thought of an early morning swim appealed to her, especially as the pool was completely devoid of other swimmers. Ten minutes later, dressed in her new swimming costume, she dived in and spent the next hour swimming up and down and thoroughly enjoying herself. When she got tired of swimming she would float on her back and enjoy the leafy branches of the trees which surrounded the perimeter. Someone had strung coloured lights through them which would have lit them attractively at night. Felicity glanced at the large clock on the side of the hotel next to the pool and decided her time of solitary enjoyment was probably coming to an end. There was no chance of meeting her mother or the slime at this hour of the morning. They would be sleeping it off, or sleeping with one another, or just plain sleeping. Besides, breakfast was calling. She retrieved her passkey from her folded towel, shook the soft white cotton out straight and threw it around her shoulders. She could smell the dining room from here. Bacon and eggs were calling.

※ ※ ※

Felicity's conjecture concerning her mother and the slime was only half correct. The slime was still unconscious in bed, her mother halfway to her audition before her daughter was out of the pool. She arrived at the audition along with a large number of other applicants. Rachel, eyeing them off warily, hoped the director was gunning for talent rather than body shape. Some of her rivals were younger and better endowed, and had dressed to suit the latter possibility. An hour passed, then two. Someone came out and told the remaining hopefuls they should go and come back after lunch at around three o'clock. Rachel left with a heavy heart, knowing that phrase often meant don't come back at all. She wandered around the building until she found a cafeteria, and managed to drink a coffee and a eat a small piece of baklava, feeling very miserable.

Three o'clock saw her back among the much smaller crowd of hopefuls in the waiting room. Apparently some of the others had interpreted the delay the same way she had almost done, and were off drowning their sorrows in something or someone. It was six o'clock before she was finally admitted into the audition room, and by that time her anxiety had given way to simmering rage. How dare they keep her waiting the whole day. Perhaps it was this attitude which gave her the edge over her rivals, because two hours later she emerged, her eyes shining, her face glowing, her heart racing as it had not done in many a day. The part was hers. There had been paperwork to sign, people to see, details to be taken down. She had been given a useful advance in salary and told to report to Universal Studios LA in one month's time. Shooting would begin in six weeks. Rachel caught a taxi back to the hotel by stepping in front of it and waving her arms. She would tell Roger first. After all, it was because of him she had an audition in the first place. Then she would tell Felicity.

Many years before she arrived at this decision, a mathematician by the name of Edward Lorenz had suggested, in terms of chaos theory, that a butterfly flapping its wings at just the right place and at just the right time, could bring about a hurricane in the weeks which followed. In Rachel's case, this small and seemingly inconsequential choice was to have much the same result.

Rachel flew up to their room only to find all Roger's clothes lying scattered on the floor and the room empty. Initially the sight caused her to think of other less pleasant possibilities. She glanced at the empty bed and went to check in the bathroom. Then it hit her – he was in the swimming pool, of course he was, how stupid she had been. Quickly rummaging through her own clothes she found her swimming costume, flung a towel around her shoulders and headed in that direction.

True to her conjecture, Roger was stroking strongly when she came bursting onto the scene, shouting and waving at him. He reached the far end of the pool and climbed out in time catch her as she flung herself into his arms, squealing with delight. "I got it, Roger. I'm off to LA. All because of you!"

The passionate kiss which followed was but prelude to the main event. Roger slipped his hands inside her bikini.

Rachel made him pause. "Roger," she said breathlessly. "There's too much light. Those coloured globes. People up there in the hotel could see us. I don't want any bad publicity—"

STORM DANCING

Roger was the sort of man who wanted it the instant his passion was aroused, as it was right now. Relinquishing her bikini he grabbed a plastic chair, and hurled it high into the string of lights. There was a popping sound and the lights went out. He returned to the bikini. "You were saying?"

"On the chaise lounge, quick."

The darkness around the pool might have prevented anyone in their apartments above from seeing anything, but they would have had to be deaf and stupid not to know what was going on. A short time later the two lovers replaced their clothing and headed up to their room, all thought of Felicity forgotten. The night manager, whose task it was to turn the pool lights off before midnight, stared out into the darkness and concluded, quite reasonably, that someone else had done it before him.

❈ ❈ ❈

The next morning Felicity headed down to the pool for another quiet, uninterrupted swim. She folded her towel as usual, placed her room passkey inside, and walked to the water's edge. A sound made her glance towards the far end of the pool. Another guest was coming for a swim. Felicity swore softly under her breath and sought refuge under the nearest poolside tree, not noticing the broken coloured glass. She didn't notice the prongs from the shattered light bulb either, until both of them stuck into her forehead. The electric current passing through her brain contracted her throat into a scream and her legs into a mighty leap. The other guest heard the scream and looked up to see a girl flying through the air. A split second later she landed in the water with an enormous splash, which died away leaving her body still and lifeless. The guest sprinted the length of the pool and jumped into the water beside her, holding her face above the surface and dragging her towards the edge. It was quite an effort to shove her over the paved lip, but he managed it. Hardly a minute had passed. The girl was breathing. He felt the pulse in her neck. There were no signs of injury, yet she was still unconscious. Perhaps she had hit her head when she fell into the pool? No, he was sure she hadn't. What had caused the scream and the leap in the first place? His first thought was a snake, and he looked quickly towards the tree, expecting to see one curled around its branches. That's when he noticed the prongs of the broken light bulb still attached to the string, then the broken glass on the paved poolside under the tree.

"Good grief, she's been electrocuted," he screamed. "Help! Help! Somebody call an ambulance. Quick."

The shouting brought other people running from the hotel. Within half an hour the girl was in an ambulance heading for the Gold Coast Hospital in Southport on siren. Police Sergeant David Green had photographed the lethal light bulb and was discussing matters with the day manager John Manning, and the man who had rescued the girl, a Mr. Frank Cubbins, on holiday with his wife who was still blissfully asleep in their apartment.

"Do we know who the girl is?" Green asked, taking another photograph with his mobile phone.

"We found her passkey wrapped up in her towel," Manning replied warily. "She's Felicity Demarra. Her mother is staying with another guest, one Roger Harman. They haven't been informed yet."

"Mother and daughter were staying separately?" Green said, surprised, pocketing his mobile phone.

"It appears that way," Manning muttered.

"Why weren't these lights reported damaged and turned off?"

"I have no idea," Manning answered in a worried voice. "You'll have to ask the duty manager who was on last night, Sam Ballard. Perhaps the string was broken and he didn't notice. We turned the other lighting off so the pool would be lit with the coloured string. We found the guests like soft pool lighting at night."

"Can you account for the breakage?" Green asked. "Something hit this bulb for it to shatter like that. The string has been placed too low in any case. Someone is going to take this hotel to the cleaners."

"I can make no comment," Manning replied defensively. "The girl might have made a full recovery by now. I'm sure we can organise some suitable compensation with her mother. A couple of nights in the hotel at our expense."

"You'd better hope so," Green said with a grimace. "Smells like negligence to me. Now, Mr. Cubbins, is it? I'd like to take a formal statement. You say you heard a scream and next you saw a girl who turns out to be Miss Demarra in the air?"

Half an hour later the duty manager knocked on Mr. Harman's door to deliver the news. Roger was barely conscious. Rachel threw some clothes over her body, and grabbing a pair of shoes in one hand and her handbag in the other, followed the manager out of the room and into the waiting taxi he had ordered in anticipation. *Do everything to show the guest the hotel is helpful, understanding and cooperative,* he thought, and then perhaps this woman wouldn't sue the pants off them for negligence.

His next stop was back at the pool area to find out why there were guests still swimming in the water. Where were the 'pool closed' signs? They had been ordered, but they hadn't come. What was happening now? A child had just cut his foot on some broken glass that hadn't been swept up properly. The manager groaned. They were going to the cleaners, no doubt about it.

Rachel Demarra flew out of the taxi and into the hospital's intensive care unit, only to learn her daughter was currently undertaking magnetic resonance imaging. No, she hadn't shown any signs of returning to consciousness, and the Registrar, in consultation with the hospital's neurosurgeon, had ordered a battery of tests. If Ms. Demarra would care to wait an hour or so...

Ms. Demarra said she would. She sat down in the waiting room feeling the mess she looked. For starters she had missed out on breakfast. It had all been too much. First the fantastic news of her audition success, then the fabulous night of passion which had followed, beginning at the pool, and now this. What had the stupid girl been doing to electrocute herself? Someone was going to pay. Other grim possibilities passed through her mind. Supposing Felicity didn't recover, or her recovery took months? She had to be in LA in four weeks or she would lose the part. No, Felicity was strong, she would recover. She had to. Then she thought of the girl herself. Was she in pain? No, she was unconscious. Thank goodness. A couple of nights to recover would mean a couple more nights with Roger, perhaps more than a couple.

Time passes slowly when you have nothing much to occupy your mind, and eventually Rachel left the waiting room, found a cafeteria in another building and bought herself a coffee and croissant. She rang Roger several times, but received no answer. The front desk had shown great reluctance to send someone up to his room, but eventually they had done so and Roger had rung back. He was sorry to hear about Felicity, but he was sure she would be alright. He had heard of film crew being electrocuted when they were shooting scenes in the rain, and they had recovered. Why didn't Rachel come back to the hotel and wait there? They could have breakfast together. Rachel considered this possibility and said she would ring him back. If there was no news from the ICU she would join him in half an hour for breakfast. There wasn't and so she did. After all, no point in waiting around when there's nothing to do, is there?

After breakfast she went to see the duty manager to find out what had happened. The tongue-in–cheek replies she received to her questions convinced her the hotel was initiating some sort of cover up.

Police sergeant Green had been more forthcoming when she had winkled his name out of the duty manager under threat of instant legal action, and by the time Roger came to take her to lunch she had the complete picture. The hotel had been negligent, creating a hazardous situation into which her poor daughter had unwittingly walked and been electrocuted. Sounded like pay dirt to her. She rang her father's firm in Sydney. Yes, they were interested. Then she rang the hospital. The neurosurgeon had been trying to contact her and sounded annoyed. Why hadn't she left a number? She was upset. Would she care to come and discuss her daughter with him? Yes she would.

That afternoon Rachel, with Roger beside her, was ushered into a small office on the first floor of the hospital. Doctor William Travers beckoned them to chairs and sat down at his desk.

He drew a folder from the bookshelf behind him and opened it. "Mr. and Mrs. Demarra—"

"Only Ms. Demarra. My name is Roger Harman, I'm just a supporting friend," Roger hastened to correct him.

Travers nodded. "Ms. Demarra, I'm afraid I have some very bad news for you." He pushed a black and white image across the table towards her. "Your daughter has sustained severe brain damage. It's not as though her brain was deprived of oxygen, as it would have been if she had not been rescued from drowning so quickly. The electric current has damaged several sections of what are called her pre-frontal areas, which is why she hasn't returned to consciousness. You can see these areas on the image."

He pointed to the sheet but Rachel wasn't even watching.

"But she will return to consciousness, won't she?" Rachel stammered, fear etched on her face. "Does she have to have all these pre-frontal things to function? I heard the human brain has lots of spare capacity, and she is a very bright child."

"There is every possibility Felicity will never return to consciousness, and if she does I'm afraid she will be severely impaired," Travers said gravely.

"Explain severely impaired," Rachel asked in a frightened voice.

"She will probably present with severe mental retardation. She will be unable to learn very much, but with patience and the correct care she might regain sufficient to enable her to take her place in some sheltered workshop. I'm afraid this accident is going to take a heavy toll on your life, Ms. Demarra."

Rachel could feel the colour draining out of her face. Her hands felt cold. How could this have happened, just when she was on the verge of being discovered by the world? Once you turned down an offer like that you never got another. How could she cope with a severely handicapped child? She knew she couldn't care for Felicity and be an actress at the same time.

She turned to Roger and laid her hand on his arm. "What am I to do?"

Roger, sensing the approaching stench of commitment, smiled like the great actor he was and squeezed her hand. "It'll be okay, Rachel. Felicity will wake up and be alright. She might be a bit slower than usual, but hey, that's an advantage, isn't it? She was always giving you a hard time. Now she's probably going to be all quiet and cooperative for a change. It will all work out for the best, you'll see."

"I would suggest you listen to more informed counsel, Ms. Demarra," Dr. Travers continued, sizing Harman up instantly. "Your friend's optimism is quite understandable but quite ridiculous. You must accept the truth, Ms. Demarra. Your daughter, if she recovers consciousness, will most certainly be intellectually as well as physically incapacitated to the point where you may even have to feed her like a baby."

It was being cruel, he knew, but he had to make a point. The stupid woman was likely to listen to the ravings of her boyfriend. Not that he would be hanging around for very long. Types like him headed off into the sunset at the slightest whiff of self-sacrifice, and this wasn't the slightest whiff. Rachel pressed her head into Roger's chest and sobbed. Life was so unfair, first her father and now this. What had she done to deserve it? Nothing. Dr. Travers showed them out of the room, enquiring if Ms. Demarra would like to see her daughter.

If she had told the truth she would have said no.

Felicity was lying on her back in a bed in the neurological ward. A feed tube filled with white liquid protruded from her nose and ran up to a large bag covered with a light-proof yellow hood. A heart monitor beeped periodically, a green light pulsed from a blood oxygen meter, a catheter tube led from under the blanket to a jar sitting on the floor, half filled with urine. Apart from these abnormal additions the girl looked exactly the same as she did when Rachel went into her bedroom each morning to wake her up. Gingerly she extended one hand and wiggled her daughter's arm. It was warm and soft and moved under her touch without resistance. She should have woken up. She didn't. Not one flicker of her eyes, not one twitch of a muscle.

'Felicity, can you hear me?" Rachel's voice was sharp, a mixture of disbelief and fear.

"She can't hear you, Ms. Demarra," Travers said quietly. "I know this is distressing for you, but Felicity is not in any pain. That is at least something you should be thankful for."

"Yes, of course, and I am, Doctor," Rachel lied.

She didn't feel thankful at all. Roger took her back to their apartment. He didn't have the heart to ask for sex that night, which showed just how deeply he had been affected by the day's events. The next day the general manager of the hotel came to see her and offered her totally free accommodation and meals while her daughter remained in hospital at Southport. There had been a staff meeting that very morning, and this response was the outcome. Perhaps the immediate investment of free hospitality would prevent further action. Rachel accepted with tearful gratitude. Their generosity was tantamount to admitting negligence. She phoned her father's law firm again. Yes, they had contacted Mr. Cubbins and were delighted to take the case, if nothing else to honour her father, a most worthy gentleman.

Two days of regular visits to his comatose daughter was more than Roger, the supportive friend, could take. The next morning he announced he was leaving for the States on the eleven o'clock plane, even though he really wanted to stay and be a support to the woman and child he loved. There had been a short argument concerning the truthfulness of this empty rhetoric, but he had left nonetheless, leaving Rachel feeling practically suicidal. She didn't even say good-bye to him. He promised faithfully to arrange a pad for them in LA when she arrived – without Felicity, of course. Air travel would no doubt be detrimental to her unstable mental condition, and he knew Rachel wouldn't want that.

Three weeks passed by. Rachel phoned Universal and was told the deadline could be extended by one week, after which they would search for another actress. Every evening she would sit at her daughter's bedside staring at her, begging her, crying and sometimes swearing at her. All the time Felicity lay there unmoving, unresponsive to her mother's pleas and insults.

Three days remained to the deadline. Pleading calls for a small extension fell on deaf ears. Either she turned up, or they got someone else. Rachel felt like screaming. She sat at her daughter's bed that evening an angry and disillusioned woman. "Why?" she screamed out loud. "Why are you doing this to me? You just lie there mocking me, smashing my life to pieces. You're going to destroy me, you know that? I wish you were dead. I wish you were dead!"

She burst into tears. At first she didn't hear the softly spoken voice of the man who had just come into the room. "May I help you?"

She glanced up and saw a stranger standing there in a white gown. He was studying the chart on the end of Felicity's bed and frowning. Rachel responded by bursting into tears again.

"Her brain's damaged," she sobbed. "She won't wake up. If she does she'll be a vegetable." She sobbed into the bedspread. "I'm her mother and I wish she was dead. She wouldn't want to live like a vegetable. I know she wouldn't." She turned towards the stranger. "You must think I'm a ghoul." More tears flooded the bedspread.

The stranger came over and put his arm gently around her shoulder. "I may be able to help you".

"And who are you?" Rachel asked defensively. "How would you possibly be able to help me? Have you any idea what I'm going through? My whole life is a ruin. A ruin! I'm supposed to be on set for a major motion picture in LA the day after tomorrow. If I don't turn up they'll get someone else, and it will be back to playing garbage in front of drug addicts."

She turned and sobbed into his shirt, allowing him to rub her back in a comforting manner. After a while she stopped, suddenly aware she was blubbing all over a complete stranger who was offering her physical comfort. She pushed herself away.

Storm Dancing

The stranger took his cue and moved respectfully to the end of the bed. "My name is Doctor Ferris," he explained. "I'm a neurologist. Doctor Travers is on another shift and I'm doing the rounds of the neurological cases, which right now amounts to only one. You are very distressed. I think I can help you best by offering you a good cup of coffee. In my profession I deal with neurological symptoms – including pain and its cure. I believe a good beverage might assist the pain you're feeling right now."

"The hospital coffee is poison, so no, thank you," Rachel sniffed.

'I wasn't thinking of hospital coffee, I was thinking of coffee at the Beach House down the road. They make a better brew. I don't think Felicity is going to wake up while you take a breather. You certainly need it."

Rachel regarded him suspiciously. It was nearly a pick up line, yet his hospital coat had Dr. D. Ferris engraved on the name tag, and he was an older man, not the sort who tried to pick up a younger woman grieving for herself at her daughter's bedside.

"You're being very kind to a stranger," she said distrustfully.

"I'm actually treating a patient, well the mother of a patient. I would ask you to believe I'm not trying to pick you up and using bereavement as a tool in my despicable game."

He smiled. There was something in his face which made Rachel believe him. Standing up, she gathered her handbag from the bed and followed him out of the room.

At 3:35 a.m. that morning Felicity Demarra died.

Dr. Ferris signed the death certificate and rang Rachel. Would she like him to arrange transfer of her daughter's body back to Sydney for cremation? Yes she would.

❋ ❋ ❋

The next day there was a short ceremony at Northern Suburbs crematorium, attended by all of three people, Rachel, some social worker or other, and the celebrant, or whatever you called the woman who pushed the button. Five hours later Ms. Rachel Demarra was on a plane heading to LA, her heart a whirlpool of conflicting emotions.

The strongest one was relief.

The film turned out to be a modest success, and eighteen months later, as a result of an out of court settlement, Ms. Demarra received a one-off payment of seven hundred and fifty thousand dollars compensation for the loss of her daughter due to negligence. Her rise to fame had begun in earnest.

Chapter 11

Storm made her way over to the dinner table on her crutches, sat down, and parked them neatly behind her chair. The rest of the family were already there. Basa transferred the large crock pot of curry onto the heat proof mat in the centre. A pile of pappadams, which Peter had enjoyed frying, occupied a dish to the right, and another tray of curry-type condiments lay to the left.

"I'm a para-plee-jick. I can't walk," Storm said triumphantly. "I learnt another word."

Peter groaned. "And guess who taught her that?"

"I did," Ellen beamed. "So now I can make another cross."

"Well she's not," Basa said crossly. "She's a little bit crippled in one leg. You used the wrong word, Ellen."

"Pree-co-shus. Ellen is pree-co-shus. I used another word," Storm continued happily.

"And guess who taught her that one?" Ellen scowled at Peter.

"Touché," Peter laughed. "Now I can make a cross too."

The crosses were three rows short of the top line of boxes. It wasn't going to be too long before the promised outing to Animal World took place. Ellen was looking forward to it. Storm was apprehensive, but didn't know how to tell anyone. Andrew and Basa had been amazed at the speed at which the latest member of their family had picked up new words and could demonstrate her understanding of them. Only two months had passed since they had started the competition, and Storm's language had improved with her vocabulary to the point where you were able to have a simple conversation without any echolalia. You could always tell when she didn't understand, because she would give you your sentence back exactly the way you said it, which was very helpful.

Peter was heavily into his studies and emerged less and less from his bedroom. Storm had sensed her new parents' disapproval when she went in there and lay down on his bed to watch him, and so she hardly ever did, although why they would object was a complete mystery to her. Not that she was bored, there was so much to see and do. Her favourite pastime was going out into the garden and drawing what she found there.

Basa, an armful of fresh clothes in her hand, knocked on the door of Storm's bedroom, and receiving no reply, went in. She put the clothes down on Storm's bed.
Artwork of various sorts was stacked up in piles near the desk in the corner. Basa went over and leafed her way through the latest A3 sketch pad which lay open on the wooden surface.

There was a whole page of lizards, tiny versions of which were likely to wind up on the walls anytime soon. Another page displayed butterflies of various shapes, drawn resting on top of tomatoes in the veggie garden. *Laying eggs I expect*, Basa thought to herself. Over the page a couple of birds were sketched without very much detail, probably because they hadn't stayed still for the artist. She turned back a few sheets and blinked in surprise.

Storm had drawn parts of herself, her hand, the musculature in her leg, a picture of her toes. Not just the outline, but in large detail, each joint carefully and accurately depicted. A medical student could have done no better. On the previous page were more drawings of the same type. In fact Storm had drawn every part of her body which was visible to her own eyes without looking in the mirror. The detail was amazing. She closed the sketch pad. *And this is the girl you wanted to send back to a sheltered workshop,* she thought to herself. A new world was opening up before Storm's eyes, and the girl was absorbing it, loving it, sucking its life into herself with joyful fascination. About the only thing she had shown a dislike of was the television, something which surprised Basa no end. Ellen whinged if she didn't get her hour each day and two on the weekend. Storm would leave the room when it was turned on.

The five hundredth word arrived on Wednesday night.

Storm proudly put the two words Andrew had taught her the day before into a sentence. "There are lots of *neurons* in our brains and they are *connected* so we work properly. That's right, isn't it, Dad?"

"Yes, Storm," Andrew said. "That's why you have trouble with your right leg. There's some bad connections in your brain. It's possible to make new connections which override the wrong ones."

"Which override the wrong ones?" Storm's eyes were large and questioning.

"Stupid of me," Andrew said. "Sorry. We have to teach your brain to make right connections, then you can use your leg properly."

"Does it hurt?" Once again the large eyes.

"Not at all, but it might make you tired."

"I'm a cripple. I don't mind." Storm shook her head determinedly. "I don't want new connections."

"You're making new connections all the time, Storm," Basa encouraged. "Whenever you draw something different, see something new, hear a different word, a new sound, your brain makes new connections. When you remember what you saw or heard your brain uses those connections to give you back the memory."

Storm looked very sad after that and said nothing for the rest of the meal, which was very unlike her. At last everyone had finished eating and the table had been cleared away. Ellen went to watch a show on TV, and Peter went back to his study. Basa put her feet up on the lounge with a book. Andrew came and stood next to Storm, who had parked herself on a kitchen chair next to her crutches.

"What's the matter?" He rubbed her on the shoulder affectionately. "Something's making you sad, so don't try to pretend."

"Pretend, make as if something is not true."

"Yes, now what's the matter?"

All of a sudden she began to cry, softly, as if she was trying to stop and was cross with herself for not succeeding. Andrew came close and put one of his arms around her shoulder. Storm turned her face into his chest and snuggled in there until she had regained control.

She lifted her large, tear-filled eyes to Andrew's face. "Dad, what was me? All I have in here" – she touched her forehead – "is new connections. What happened to all the others? I know babies begin very small. There are pictures of them in books. But I'm not small. I didn't start small, but I must have. What was me?"

It was a long time before Andrew answered. "Storm, whatever you were is somehow lost. I don't know why or how. I don't think we will ever know why or how. The only thing that matters is who you are now, and that we love you."

"You mightn't."

"What do you mean?" Andrew stroked her hair softly.

"If you find out why or how. You mightn't."

"Are you afraid we mightn't?"

Storm Dancing

Storm nodded her head then shook it. Two big tears rolled down her cheeks. "I mightn't. I mightn't like me. I don't want any old connections to what I was. I don't want to know."

Andrew folded the girl in his arms and held her close. How to answer in some way which was half convincing? There was an element of truth in what she feared.

"Storm, there's a little bit of the same fear in all of us, me included," he said comfortingly. "There are things in my past which I'm not proud of. I don't want to remember them because I'm ashamed, if you really want to know, but I can't change them. What matters is the way I live now. We're not perfect."

"We're not perfect?" Storm lifted her lovely eyes to his face again.

"We all have bits that aren't right, aren't good," Andrew explained. "A perfect person is someone who has no bad bits."

"Who's perfect?"

"Nobody." Andrew continued to stroke her hair.

"I want to be."

"Oh, Storm," Andrew sighed. "I wish that was possible, but nobody is ever going to be perfect. Whatever you were, you have become the way you are, Storm. If anything of your before life comes back we will still love you, even if it's all bad. It's what you're like now that matters, not how you were once upon a time."

"I was in a dark, dark place of no love, and I came here," Storm shuddered. "How did I come here?"

Andrew tightened his arms around the girl. "I haven't the faintest idea. You came with the storm, that's all I know."

"Some... some... I don't know word... some big, big power... did it 'cause he wanted me here."

"Perhaps you're trying to say God wanted you here."

"Who is God?" Storm's eyes seemed to have grown in size.

Andrew laughed softly. "That's far too big a question for tonight, young lady. I'm not sure I can answer it in any case. Do you know, I don't think we'll wait for the next five hundred words. I think you know enough for us to start helping you to walk."

Fear filled Storm's eyes again. "I don't want to make walking connections. Don't want to go away."

Andrew laughed and hugged her tightly. "We won't send you away if you can walk properly, Storm. What a ridiculous idea. You're part of our family now. We all love you very much. Don't you realise that?"

"Don't ... *deserve* ... that is the right word? Don't deserve. I'd be dead if you didn't love me, Daddy."

She hugged him tightly, which was just as well, because Andrew would have had some trouble answering her right then. He held her until he felt her arms relax a little and kissed her on top of her head.

Struggling to keep his voice normal, he released the girl and picked up her crutches. "Would you like to see what Peter is doing in his room? He needs a distraction. The boy has been studying too hard lately."

"I'm a distraction?" Storm raised her eyebrows.

"You're one enormous, lovely distraction."

Storm smiled at him, reached up and kissed his cheek. Taking the crutches from his hand, she set off for Peter's room. She wasn't sure what a distraction was, but she rather liked the thought of being one. She opened Peter's door without knocking, came in and curled up on the bed.

STORM DANCING

"Dad says you need a distraction – me."

Peter threw down the pen he was writing with and rubbed his eyes with the back of his hands. "Dad said that?" He laughed. "Tell you what, I'll read you a story if you like. Do you want to pick one?"

An hour later Basa came into the room to tell her son it was time to stop studying and go to sleep. She found the two of them sound asleep, Storm curled up on the bed with her head on Peter's chest. At first she wondered if she should leave them that way, but in the end woke the girl up gently and helped her move quietly back to her own room.

❀ ❀ ❀

The next day was unseasonably hot.

Ellen had a pupil free day. Being somewhat at a loss for things to do with Peter at school and Mum and Dad at work, she decided to capitalise on the discomfort of everyone else by running a lemonade stand at the garage down the road, and conscripted Storm into helping. Ellen explained how the lemonade had to be made with lots of sugar and lemons from the tree in the backyard stirred in with water and finally ice cubes. They would use paper cups to avoid washing up, and a cooler bag to carry the cold juice. She commissioned Storm to draw a picture of someone pouring a cup of lemonade down their throat and put the words 'so refresing 20¢ a glass' on it in big letters. The picture was fine, but Ellen had to do the letters. She spelled 'refreshing' wrong, but in the scheme of things it probably added to the effect.

"Why will people come in here to get this drink?" Storm said without enthusiasm. "Mum will not like this picture on the wall."

"They don't come in here, stupid," Ellen snorted. "We go to the garage down the road. The man who owns it is a patient of Dad's and he'll be helpful or I'll say Dad is thinking of sending him to another doctor."

"That's a pretend, isn't it?" Storm frowned her annoyance.

"No, it's a lie. I'm good at it. Come on, it will take a couple of trips. Here's a rope you can attach to your crutch – unless you want to try dancing down there."

"Not dancing," Storm retorted angrily. "You want me to help you won't say dancing. Crippled. You don't understand."

Ellen made her usual lightning assessment of Storm's mood and concluded another joke like that would result in her doing the lot herself. "Sorry," she said quickly. "Come on, I'll tie the rope to the side of the card table. You put the sticky tape and picture in this plastic bag."

It took three trips to the garage to do it. One to get the table down there, one to carry the lemonade and table cloth, and one to get the cups which they had forgotten, along with some small change from Ellen's money box. Annette the secretary had poked her nose in and made some disparaging comment about a complete waste of time, so no doubt Andrew would know what was going on by now. Storm discovered that crutches are great to get around on and hopeless for carrying tables and large cooler bags of lemonade. The more she struggled with the load the more she began to think these new connections in her head might just be worth it. The owner of the garage had suggested a place in the shade over near the 'Air and Water' but not in front of it, and got one of the mechanics to sticky tape the sign high up on the wire fence behind it.

Ellen noticed the young man was taking a fair amount of interest in Storm and hardly noticing her. Corrective measures had to be applied. "When people come over, make sure you have those crutches on and look tired and crippled," Ellen said, spreading the paper cups out on the table.

"I am tired and crippled," Storm said unhappily. "Why can't I sit down on the chair your friend has brought? There's two of them."

"It would distract customers. You see it's not just the lemonade that does it, you have to look cute," Ellen told her with a confidential air. "You stare into their faces and smile. Then you say "would you like some of my refreshing lemonade?" If they go to turn away you put on a really unhappy face, like this."

She changed her face into such a sad expression it made Storm laugh. "But you don't want me to sit down and look cute, you want me to stand up all the time and be crippled," she complained.

"Exactly. Sitting down you look – too cute. That boy from the garage will be mewing around here all the time and driving the customers away. If he comes over and asks you out, say 'thanks but no thanks.' Can you do that?"

"Thanks but no thanks," Storm frowned. "Silly. Yes and no together."

"Say it anyway, I'll get Mum to explain later."

The lemonade stand was a fiscal success. Four times Storm had to go back to the house and make more lemonade, leaving Ellen playing 'cute' and collecting the money. When the time came for them to pack up and go home she was feeling very tired indeed, and quite looking forward to making a whole lot of new brain connections. All in all they had collected twenty dollars, ten from selling lemonade and ten from a man who had come over and bought the picture Storm had drawn, which made Ellen very cross.

"What a waste of time," Ellen grumbled as they made their second trip home with the table banging annoyingly against Storm's crutches. "We could have done so much better if we had just sold your drawings and given them a free cup of lemonade while they flipped through them. I suppose I'll have to give you half the money now, less my commission, of course."

"Keep it," Storm said wearily. "What would I do with money?"

"You're so naïve."

"What's naïve?"

"Innocent. You don't know how the world works."

"I like innocent," Storm said. "You're not innocent, are you?"

"Innocent is for the birds!" Ellen snapped.

Innocent she may have been, but it didn't take Storm very long to figure out that little girls got cranky when they were very tired.

CHAPTER 12

James Hunt completed his degree in journalism with a list of high distinctions in nearly every subject. The faculty at The University of Technology Sydney had offered him honours with the possibility of even further study, but he had opted to go into the workforce. It was purely a coincidence that a major Sydney newspaper laid off around two thousand staff the very day he went to them for a job. The instability in what one would have thought an ever burgeoning industry, had the effect of closing almost every door which James had assumed would be flung wide when he presented his excellent credentials.

He had tried freelance, but nobody was willing to pay for the articles he prepared. His parents had decided to spend their children's inheritance and moved up to a retirement villa at Port Macquarie, two minutes amble from fine white sands and crystal blue water. Good luck to them. By now his funds were running low, and in desperation he had answered an advertisement from the editor of a metropolitan regional newspaper, the Northern Voice. A week later the man had offered him a very junior position on the staff with a salary to match. James had accepted, feeling the need to eat and pay the rent. The job was unrelenting dreariness, and he thought if he wrote one more article about another domestic animal rescued from some horrible fate he would go completely nuts.

His editor, George McGuiness, reminded him of those Neanderthal specimens he had seen in picture books, and James felt with certain justification the man had a brain to match his appearance. Whenever he caught the whiff of a decent story, George would give it to someone else, or tell him to drop the investigation. A certain mayor was often seen in the company of a prominent politician's eye-candy wife. "Coincidence," George said. "Back off." The local council spent twenty million dollars on some worthless real estate worth a tenth of the price. "Nobody's interested in that sort of muck raking," George said. A woman had found six Siamese kittens in a water pipe. "Go for it," George said, "front page stuff. Make sure you get a photograph of her holding a kitten, the readers loved pictures like that." James often thought a good exposé on George himself would be worth doing, but there wasn't an interested paper he could sell it to. Sometime after that he would be found dead in a rubbish bin. George carried a certain air of menace as he strode around the office blasting a compositor here and a reporter there.

It was hot, very hot.

The office air conditioning had never worked well, almost certainly due to George's unwillingness to spend a cent on it, and now it had given up the ghost completely. It was making a loud grating sound which carried through the ducting into every corner of the office. The racket, combined with the heat and the sound of George's raving, was enough to reduce a reasonable man to the verge of quivering insanity. He glanced up from the article he was writing on inadequate drainage. Sally Lyons in the cubicle opposite him was trying to stuff rubbers into her ears. Failing in the attempt to mute the racket, she swiped her keyboard towards the rubbish bin. Now it was hanging by its cable off the end of her desk, swinging from side to side. *Time to go,* James thought to himself, *before I end up completely round the twist.* He hit return and sent the article to the editor's desk, turned off the computer and headed out towards the car park. His Toyota had been mercifully parked in the shade, but even so the steering wheel was so hot he could hardly bear to touch it.

By the time he had reached Shepherd's Bush Drive in Cherrybrook not far from where he lived, the car air conditioning had brought the interior and its occupant back to a sensible temperature. James glanced at the fuel gauge and decided he needed to fill up. Swinging the vehicle off the road into a garage, he noticed some kids had set up a lemonade stand near the 'Air and Water' service against the rear fence. Above them someone had drawn a picture. James had a sister who was an artist, and through her he had become interested in art himself. He parked his car in the bay, opened the petrol cap, shoved the nozzle from the pump into the hole, and the petrol cap into the filler handle so he didn't have to sit there while the tank filled up. He walked over to the lemonade stand. Two girls were there, a teenager on crutches who seemed tired, and a younger one sitting on a chair looking fed up. He watched the expression on her face change as he approached.

"Would you like some of our refreshing lemonade?" the younger one said with a beguiling smile.

How could he resist? James took out twenty cents from his pocket and held his hand out for the cup. He had other interests in mind, however. "Did you draw the picture?" he asked.

"No, my sister did." Ellen pointed to the girl on the crutches. "She's a paraplegic, always in a lot of pain. We're raising money to get her some special treatment in the United States."

The older girl turned round to her sister and glared at her. "She pretends a lot. I drew the picture," she said with a smile.

"Would you sell it to me for ten dollars?" James asked.

"Yes, she would." The younger girl was instantly on her feet. "That would help with the doctor's bills. They're so expensive. Our parents work their fingers to the bone but it isn't enough."

Another glare from the older girl.

"I can't get it down," the teenager said, apologetically. "Sorry. Can you? We're finishing up now. That was the last lemonade. It was warm. Sorry."

"I'd be delighted to, James said. "I notice you haven't signed your name on it. Can you do that?"

He fetched the picture down, and before Ellen had a chance to stop her, Storm had taken up the pen the stranger held out to her and began to write on the bottom "S t o r..." She had seen Peter write her name and knew how to do it.

Ellen snatched the pen out of her hand. "Stor is short for Stornway, our family name before we changed it when we came to Australia many years ago."

"How fascinating," James smiled. "Tell me, Miss Stornway, would you like a nice drink of cold lemonade? I would be happy to buy you one while you tell me where you learned to draw like that."

He noticed the younger girl's foot had come to rest on top of Miss Stornway's and was pushing down hard.

"Thanks but no thanks," Storm replied.

"Are you sure?"

"No, it's what I'm supposed to say. I don't know what it means."

James stared at her, trying to work out if she was making fun of him, and decided she wasn't. There was something strange about the girl, something he couldn't put his finger on. The younger girl had rolled her eyes into the top of her head in utter disgust, but the teenage girl was smiling at him, and there was a quality of freshness in her face which he found intriguing. There was something else as well, a memory, but of what? He glanced towards the petrol pump and saw that it had finished filling the tank.

Taking a ten dollar note out of his pocket he handed it to the teenager. "Do you have any more pictures like that?" he asked with a smile. "They would sell better than warm lemonade."

He rolled the picture up carefully and headed back towards the garage store to pay for the petrol. A short time later he came out with two cans of lemonade, walked over to the girls packing up their table and handed

136

one to each of them. "Thirsty work," he laughed. "You're both hot and tired. Here's a drink, I know you need it."

The young girl grunted something and took the can without looking at him. The teenager took the other from his hand and laughed. "Thank you. I like proper lemonade."

"You're welcome." James went back to the car and started the engine. Yes, the teenage girl reminded him of someone he had seen somewhere before, not a teenager. Stornway? Why didn't the little girl want him to know her name? Perhaps because he was a stranger, but there was something more to it. No, he was beginning to imagine mysteries where there weren't any. Still, there was no doubt about the teenage girl's skill as an artist. He would show his sister when he saw her next week.

CHAPTER 13

One week after the lemonade stall the family had gone to Animal World. This explained why two ducklings – one who had arrived with a broken leg and another with an injured wing – were roaming around in a cage on the back lawn as healthy as you please. Storm was so enraptured with the animals it had been awfully difficult to get her back in the car. The young woman who was in charge of showing the children around had only released the two fluffy bundles into her care because she was almost sure they were going to die anyway. Besides, she couldn't bear the look of those big pleading eyes for much longer. There followed days of nursing and feeding and allowing them to stay on Storm's bed in a box during the night. The afternoon at Berowra Waters never eventuated.

Storm's passion for all things living extended to plants as well. There were a number of Oak trees lining the street, and since Storm learned that the small smooth brown egg-shaped things littering the footpath were acorns, there were a number of young Oak seedlings growing in the back yard under the most careful attention. There were bean seeds growing in cotton wool, rose stems sprouting in jars, and Petunias planted in neat rows under the window sills.

"She has a passion for life the like of which I've never encountered," Andrew said to Basa as they watched their charge sprinkling the garden with a fine water spray. "I've never seen our backyard look so green and growing."

On the Sunday after their extended visit to Animal World, Andrew put up the second page of boxes.

Storm waved her arm towards it dismissively. "I don't want to learn more words like this," she announced. "Teach me to read."

It wasn't so much a request as an ultimatum. Ellen, who was far in advance of her age in language, had shown no inclination to match her reading with her astounding vocabulary. She could write sentences and read the books from school when her teacher insisted, and found them monumentally, indescribably boring. Nothing in the family library competed with the instant entertainment on TV. Storm on the other hand, was just the opposite. She progressed through Ellen's nursery books at a slow and steady rate, simultaneously writing out the words she was being taught to read. Basa, Andrew and Peter took turns to teach, and if the girl had had her way they would have begun after breakfast and finished after dinner.

Despite Andrew's assertion the family should start training Storm to walk, five whole months went by before he had managed to construct the apparatus required to do it. The practice had become exceptionally busy, and Andrew was sometimes called out before breakfast and often on the weekends. By Sunday evening he would collapse into a comfortable chair in the lounge room and go to sleep.

Peter was now engrossed in his studies every night and most of the weekends, which Ellen didn't mind and Storm hated. Basa and Andrew had tried to explain as patiently as they could that Storm could help him by staying out of his room because she was a distraction. Storm had no idea how she could help anyone by keeping away from them, but once again her gratitude manifested itself in obedience, and she never went near Peter's bedroom door. She told him very seriously that she was a distraction, and distractions weren't good for him. Rather than coming into his room she would wait all day in the kitchen with her book until he had time to come out and teach her to read. This innocent enticement increased her power of distraction by several orders of magnitude.

Storm's training began the first week in June. Andrew's persistence had made up for whatever skill he lacked at carpentry, and he regarded his finished construction with a quiet sense of pride. The family regarded it with a quiet sense of relief. The device consisted of an ordinary flat, non-motorised treadmill. Beside it on the left, Andrew had constructed a level platform of the same height and length. At the end of the platform he had attached a vertical post. Through the post was a strong horizontal handle for Storm to hold on to while they were training her right leg.

Storm presented herself for treatment with all the enthusiasm of a dead wombat, dressed in a one piece swimming costume Basa had bought her for the purpose. She had absolutely forbidden Ellen and Peter to watch despite their protests. This was going to be bad enough without an audience.

Basa took one look at her face as she came into the garage and gave her a hug. "You're a brave young woman, Storm. Andrew – Dad - and I don't expect you to make the same sort of progress you've made with everything else. Just do your best and keep trying. We know this is hard for you."

Andrew reached out his hand and helped Storm onto the platform. "Good girl. This is called a treadmill." He demonstrated by pushing the fibre mat around with his hand. "We want you to stand on the platform with your left leg, hold on to the handle, and put your right foot on the treadmill. That's the way. Now Mum is going to hold your thigh and I am going to hold your calf and your foot. We want you to relax your leg, that's right. Now we're going to move your leg the way it should go when you walk straight. Feel the sensation. Watch closely with your eyes. We have to train your brain to rely on what your eyes are seeing, not what your muscles tell you they're doing. Feel the movement, watch it closely."

Andrew and Basa knelt down next to the treadmill and gripped Storm's leg, moving it carefully forward and down until her foot was on the treadmill, then pushing it back as if she was walking. They did this several times.

"See the movement?" Andrew asked.

"I see it." Storm said, staring down at her foot. "That's the way I tell my leg to move."

"Alright," Andrew continued, "now we want you to take a deliberate step with your right leg. This time we are going to stop your leg moving in the wrong way. Don't fight us too hard, but this time you do the moving, alright?"

"Okay."

Storm's right foot shot out across her left one, and Andrew had quite a struggle forcing the muscles to move the way they should have done.

"You stop my leg from going straight," Storm complained, attempting to wiggle free.

"Storm, watch the way your leg moves when you tell it to go straight." Andrew said, letting go while the girl moved her leg as instructed.

"It goes wrong, across the other one," Storm said, her distress rising.

"That's right," Basa said. "Now we're going to make it move straight like it should. Don't fight us too hard, but you have to do the movement. You will feel us push your leg in what might seem the wrong direction, but it's the right direction. Keep watching the way your foot moves, that's what your brain has to learn."

The session lasted half an hour. It was all Storm could take. Each time her leg refused to do what she told it she became upset. Each time they corrected her movement it felt as though they were deliberately pushing her leg the wrong way. There were tears of frustration in her eyes before they stopped, and no apparent progress had been made at all.

"That's alright, Storm. It takes time to make new connections," Andrew comforted, his arms around their tearful patient.

"We will do half an hour every day in the mornings at five a.m. before breakfast. Ellen and Peter don't mind getting the breakfast ready while we're out here. It takes the two of us to move your leg and foot muscles the way they ought to go. After a few weeks we should see a lot of improvement."

Two months came and went and the improvement was barely noticeable. Far more noticeable were Ellen's increasing protests at having to get up half an hour earlier, and Peter, whilst not complaining at all, was becoming more exhausted by the day. His HSC trial exams were in a few weeks and tomorrow he had an assessment in Physics. Much depended on that result.

❄ ❄ ❄

On Sunday night, three weeks before Peter's birthday, tragedy struck.

"Damn and blast the bloody load of shit!" Peter's angry outburst echoed down the hall, followed by some thumping, crashing sounds.

The rest of the family who were in the lounge room doing whatever, stopped doing it immediately. Peter never swore, and hardly ever raised his voice, now he had done both, loud enough for the neighbours to hear even though his bedroom door was closed. Andrew jumped up from his newspaper and headed down the hall to the bedroom, followed by Basa with Storm bringing up the rear on her crutches. Ellen decided there were quite enough people to handle the crisis, and besides, her show was nearing an exciting conclusion which she didn't want to miss. Andrew opened the door to find his son holding his head with both hands, the remains of his laptop upside down on the floor. He turned round with tears in his eyes.

"The hard drive is stuffed, he said bitterly. "I've lost an English assignment. Ten hours work. Gone."

"Backup?" Andrew said cautiously.

"Guess what, Dad, if I had a backup would I be like this? I always back up, but guess who forgot this time? Now I'll have to reload the operating system and then all the data before I can even begin the damn thing again. I don't know how I'm going to finish it on time."

Storm pushed her way to the front. "Peter... What? There are tears."

She came over to him on her crutches and wrapped her arms around his neck, obviously distressed. Basa was about to tell her to give Peter some space, but the expression on his face gave her cause for pause. Storm's embrace had taken much of the anger out of his eyes. Yes, she was calming him. Without comprehending the problem, she was calming him. Perhaps he felt he couldn't be angry when he saw she was upset? Whatever the reason it was working. A full minute passed before Peter stood up and Storm let go.

"Sorry for the language," he said, apologetically. "I reached the limit. Feel like a dork."

"I would have probably said worse," Andrew sympathised. "Use the computer in the surgery. Plug your backup drive in the USB connection at the front. If you need some stuff typed into the word processor, just dictate it into my voice recorder and Annette will do it. I'll manage the patients myself for a few hours. I think you've written off the laptop." He picked it up with one hand and its screen with the other. "Don't worry. It was pretty obsolete in any case."

"Thanks, Dad." Peter knew it wasn't, and his action had brought its obsolescence forward a considerable distance. "I lost my block and it was the closest thing around."

A short time later an earlier version of the assignment was discovered in the waste paper basket near the networked printer in the breakfast room. The discovery lifted Peter's spirits considerably, even though some of the pages were covered with the remains of egg on toast. Using these as a guide he wrote out the corrections and dictated everything into his father's machine. Annette could produce the file tomorrow and he would put the finishing touches on it that night.

The family had gone to bed, and Peter was just about to turn off the light, when he saw the door open and Storm standing in the doorway.

"Can the distraction come in?"

"Of course," Peter muttered apologetically. "Sorry about tonight, you missed a reading lesson."

The girl came over and sat down on the bed. "How much money is a lap top thing?"

"Too much. I don't want another one like that, it's very slow."

"It doesn't move very fast?" Storm frowned at him.

"It doesn't do what it's supposed to do very fast. No, when I get another one it will be a quad core i7 with all the bells and whistles."

"How much does this quad with the bells and whistles need for money?" Storm asked casually.

"More than I've got in the bank," Peter said sadly. "I'm not going to ask Dad for it either, because I wrecked a perfectly good laptop when I got angry."

"How much money?" Storm persisted.

"Fifteen hundred dollars."

"And how many tens are there in fifteen hundred?"

"One hundred and fifty. Why are you asking me this Storm?"

"Maybe I am wanting you to teach me maths."

"One day, not now." He paused, suddenly serious. "Storm, you saw me get angry and I felt ... like I let you down."

"Let me down? I was standing up," Storm frowned.

"No," Peter explained. "I behaved like a horrible person. I never want you to see how a horrible person behaves."

"You are my Protector, not a horrible person." Storm reached out and laid her hand gently on his arm.

"I wasn't tonight."

"You will always be my Protector, Peter." She leant over him and planted a kiss on his cheek. "Goodnight. The distraction is going to bed now."

She slid off the bed, picked up her crutches and left the room. Peter reached up and turned off the light, but tired as he was he couldn't manage to sleep. Storm's words echoed through his mind, "you will always be my Protector, Peter". How long was always? The answer to that question troubled him. Someday her wings would grow strong and beautiful, and she would fly away. A pain for which he had no name gripped his heart. All he knew is he never wanted that day to come.

❄ ❄ ❄

Basa had left for work, Andrew was in the surgery, and Annette was doubtless enjoying her unexpected assignment. Ellen and Storm were clearing away the breakfast things. There had been no walking practice that morning.

"Ellen," Storm said suddenly, "if you wanted to go to the Village, you know, where Mum takes us sometimes, how would you go?"

"Without Mum? Ask Dad for a lift."

"Without Mum or Dad. Say you wanted to go there by yourself without Mum or Dad to buy a present for them."

"At the Village? Happy birthday, Mum, here's a nice fresh cabbage," Ellen laughed.

"Ellen, be sensible please."

"There's a bus comes along going the opposite way just after the school bus."

"How much money does it cost?"

"Twenty five cents I think. Why are you asking? What's going on?" Ellen frowned.

"I want to explore my world a little. The Village is 'a little', isn't it?"

"Oh yeah, it's a very little Village. If you go Mum will be mad and Peter will freak out."

"Which is why you won't tell them."

"Why won't I tell them again?"

"Because I saw you stuff Mum's good table cloth under the house when you accidentally cut it with scissors."

"Deal. You're learning fast."

Ellen went back into her room to make final preparations for school, and Storm went back into her room to make some preparations of her own. She took out all the money Ellen had given her from the lemonade stall, selected a handful of it and put it in a green shopping bag. Next she tied a large ribbon around a collection of her paintings and made a loop for a handle. She heard the front door slam which meant Ellen had gone out and her bus would be coming soon. Coming into the kitchen on her crutches, she filled a plastic bottle with water, added it to the green bag and set off on her adventure. It was only a short wait for the bus. It was quite an effort to get on board with crutches while carrying all her packages, but she managed it finally and parked them on the railing next to the driver.

"How much money?" Storm asked.

"Twenty five cents Miss", the driver growled. "Can't you read?"

"Not very well."

"Don't give me any bullshit or you get off."

Storm stared at him in total confusion. She scooped out a handful of coins and handed them to the man.

"You're just plain dumb, aren't you?" he growled again. "Here, keep the rest, now go and sit down."

Storm hadn't quite managed to sit down before the driver accelerated away from the curb. She would have gone flying down the aisle were it not for a kind woman who sprang up and grabbed her by the arm.

"He's such a pig," she said. "I've a good mind to report him over this. You just sit there sweetie. Where are you going?"

"The Village. He doesn't look like a pig. He's not a nice man I think."

"You're right there."

Five minutes later with some assistance from the same kind woman, Storm was standing on the pavement outside the Village. She moved on her crutches over to a shady section of square towards the back of the supermarket, undid the ribbon around the bundle, extracted a sign which said "PICTURES $10" and stuck it up with sticky tape on the side of a used clothing bin. Yes, that was perfect. Brushing away some dead gum leaves from the pavement she spread out nine of her artworks and sat down next to them with her crutches on one side and the remainder of the bundle on the other.

The day dragged on interminably. Only a few people even noticed her there as they made their way to their cars. Others walked by in the distance as if she was invisible, no one bought a thing. Storm had nearly finished her bottle of water, and her legs were getting very stiff and sore from sitting in the one place for so long. She stood up on her crutches to ease the pain, and noticed a young man was trying very hard to open the door of a car parked under the shade of the gum trees at the far side of the car park, quite near her. Perhaps she could help. She picked up her crutches and made her way over towards him. When she was quite close the young man turned round and saw her. He grabbed the piece of tape he had been using to force the latch and ran. Storm was so taken aback she didn't watch what she was doing with her crutches, and the next minute the young man was flying through the air, only to make a most undignified landing in the middle of a row of shopping trolleys.

Events moved very swiftly after that. A man came running from the direction of the supermarket shouting "get him!" very loudly, followed by several others who must have been near their cars. They cornered the young man and grabbed hold of him. He was saying a whole lot of words Storm didn't understand, even though he said them very loudly, but the men weren't letting go. It wasn't very long before another man in a dark blue coat came up and took the young man away to an odd shaped car.

The man who had arrived first came over to Storm. "Thank you so very much, young lady," he beamed. "I'm the manager of the supermarket. We were losing custom because of that villain. What's your name?"

"Storm," she replied.

"Pretty name. You must be a very sharp young woman. How did you notice him?"

"I was selling my paintings over there." Storm pointed with her arm. "I'm sorry if I've made trouble."

"Trouble?" the manager laughed. "No way. How are sales going? May I see what you've done?"

Four of the nine paintings disappeared at once. Storm replaced them with four more. The manager went and stuck them up in the supermarket. He must have made an announcement of some kind as well, because from that time on Storm had one customer after another. An hour later she had sold the lot, and still people came over to buy.

"You're very gifted," an older woman said. "Will you be back tomorrow? I'd like our ladies group to see your work."

Storm Dancing

"I'll be back tomorrow," Storm promised.

She went into the supermarket to thank the manager. He gave her a large bottle of ice cold water because she looked hot and tired.

"You come back any time," he said. "There's a better spot just outside the store. I'll have it roped off and ready for you. I take it you're a professional artist?"

"No, I'm buying my brother a laptop because his old one broke, and it went slow. I'm not sure why it went slow, but he needs one to go faster," Storm said with large, sincere eyes.

"I take it this is a surprise?"

"Yes."

"You come back tomorrow," the manager laughed. "Tell you what, don't bring any lunch, the store will provide it. I'm going to get more customers because of you, just wait and see."

Storm came back tomorrow. By the end of the week she had a large collection of ten dollar notes and an even larger fan club at the Village. The bus from the Village was running late on Friday afternoon, and Storm arrived back at the house just after Ellen had come home. Every other day she had managed to dispose of the green bag, wash the tiredness off her face, and curl up on the lounge before the girl burst through the front door.

"Where have you been?" Ellen said suspiciously. "What's in the green bag?"

"At the Village. Why?"

"Did you go this morning too? How boring. I think I'll tell Mum."

"Remember the tablecloth."

"What do you do up there?" Ellen demanded. "Swipe food from the shop? I'm still going to tell Mum."

"And your best shoes you ruined when you played and didn't change."

"I threw them out," Ellen countered.

"I picked them up."

"Damn," Ellen snapped. "Blackmailers always come to a horrible end. Can I go into your room?"

"They're not in there."

"The police will come and arrest you for shoplifting and loitering and put you in jail," Ellen threatened angrily.

"Remember the shoes."

"I'm going to watch TV," Ellen snapped. "You're heading for big trouble."

Storm had picked the shoes out of the bin simply because she had thought they didn't belong there. There were scratches on the bright red leather and she had painted them out with bright red paint, intending to give them back to Ellen as a surprise. One day she would, in the meantime they served another useful purpose.

CHAPTER 14

The weekend passed quickly and enjoyably except for the walking lessons which Storm had learned to hate with a passion, only enduring them because of all the trouble Andrew and Basa took each time. Ellen had been sour and cranky, partly because she didn't like it when someone managed to get the better of her, and partly because she was quite worried about this new development in Storm's behaviour. In this case it was entirely justified. Storm was just Storm. What would happen if someone asked her name? She hoped the girl was as good at shoplifting as she was at painting. There was a nasty streak there which she hadn't seen before, she thought. Perhaps Storm was turning slowly but surely into an arch criminal, driven by her dark and mysterious past.

Ellen watched a great deal more TV than was good for her.

On Monday Storm went to the Village again and returned on a much earlier bus having sold all her artwork. On Tuesday she gathered up every single painting she could find and set off again. A small busload of women arrived an hour later and bought every painting she had taken with her. What to do now? There were people still coming over and wanting to see her art. An opportunity like this should not be wasted. There was a newsagency near the supermarket which sold paper and pencils. She had been there before when Basa had bought her the paper to draw on. Yes, that might work. She told the small crowd to wait, and picking up her crutches, made her way over to the shop. A little while later she emerged with a pile of A2 sized drawing paper, a pencil sharpener and a whole box of pencils.

"I'll draw you," she said. "Can you sit down on the chair?"

The chair had been provided by the manager of the supermarket who had been concerned to see the girl sitting cross-legged on the square next to her crutches for hours on end. There was some murmuring in the crowd. A few people walked away, one of the older ladies sat down in the chair.

"Draw away pet," she said. "I've nothing better to do for an hour or so. I think Harry would like a portrait of his aunt."

Storm didn't know who Harry was, but she did know that the woman had badly overestimated the necessary time. Sitting down on the square next to the pile of paper she began to draw, occasionally glancing up into the woman's face. In all of ten minutes she handed the pencil sketch to the woman, and the woman handed her twenty dollars.

"You're some gifted artist," she said, "where did you learn to draw?"

"I could draw before I could talk," Storm explained.

"Incredible!" The woman exclaimed. "I have to tell Harry about this." She stood up and went away. Another woman plonked herself down on the chair and dragged her small boy onto her lap.

"Be still, Eustace. Off you go, my dear. If you could do it as fast as the one you did for the other lady I'd appreciate it. I have to pick Suzie up from netball in half an hour."

By the end of the day Storm's wrist ached and two boxes of pencils had been reduced to small stubs. There were a large number of orange coloured notes in her bag now. She liked the colour better than the blue ones. The owner of the Village newsagency had ordered two reams of A2 drawing paper, and could they deliver it tomorrow?

Storm Dancing

On Wednesday, Harry, the nephew of the first woman she drew, came over to see her for himself. Storm noticed he was carrying a large black thing in his hand.

"Hi," he said, "I'm Harry Sloane. You drew a picture of my aunt Elizabeth yesterday. You're one heck of a talented young woman. Aunt tells me you said you could draw before you could talk?"

"Yes." Storm smiled a little shyly up at him. "I still have some trouble with talking."

"But not with drawing. You're a prodigy, a Cherrybrook celebrity. I'm from the Voice. Do you mind if I take your picture for the newspaper?"

"I don't think I'm very pretty. There are lots of better things to take pictures of."

"You're pretty enough, young woman. You don't mind? Thanks. Just sit there drawing on that piece of paper and look up, that's it. Great. Now tell me about yourself. What's your name?"

"Storm."

"Storm who?"

"Just Storm."

Ah, I see, that's your artist's name, isn't it? What's your real one?"

"Storm is my real name." Storm wrinkled her forehead. Why was this man asking stupid questions?

"Okay, okay, I get it," Harry chuckled knowingly. "Where do you live, Storm?"

"Down the road. I catch the bus. Do you catch the bus?"

"Not usually, but I might this afternoon. Let me buy you some lunch. You're going to be famous, you know that?"

MAC CUSITER

"I don't need lunch, Storm explained. "Matthew, the manager of the supermarket brings me lunch."

"Matthew, is it? I'll bet he knows when he's on to a good thing."

Storm furrowed her brow. What was this strange man saying?

"Now I'm off for a bit," Harry said. "Just another picture? Look up, smile, yeah, that's a better one."

It was a better one because from that angle, photographing Storm drawing on the ground with her head tilted up towards him, he could see a lot more of her cleavage. Readers liked cleavage, or at any rate, he did.

The customers kept coming all that afternoon, and by around two thirty Storm had mercifully run out of paper. It was Peter's birthday tomorrow, so whatever she had collected would have to do for a present. If it wasn't enough she would keep going until it was.

She caught the bus home a bit earlier that afternoon, surprised to see the man who called himself Harry get off at her stop with her.

"Can I help you across the road?" he asked.

"Thanks but no thanks," Storm replied, remembering how she was supposed to answer unwanted invitations.

"Okay," Harry smiled. "You live over there?"

"The house with the yellow fence around. It's nice, isn't it?" Storm pointed with a crutch.

"It's very nice," Harry grinned. "See you soon."

Why she should see Harry soon quite escaped her. She crossed the road, let herself into the house with the key that was always kept under the gardenia pot on the porch, and went to wash her face. No need to draw Ellen's attention to her continuing daily excursions. She knew the threat

154

of shoes and tablecloth was not going to hold forever. Never mind, she had reached her goal, or at least the first part of it. Going back into her room she gathered up all the money she had stored at the bottom of a drawer and added it to the collection already in the bag. She tied the handles together with a piece of ribbon, and drew a little card with a picture of a laptop on it, as close as she could remember from the one which had disintegrated on the floor. She knew this one had to be a faster laptop, but she didn't quite know how to make it look faster. Never mind. She hoped he would be pleased. After dinner, that was the time to give her present, before Peter became engrossed in his studies.

All through the evening meal Storm was quivering with an inexplicable air of excitement. Ellen was suspicious, Andrew and Basa amused, and Peter was too tired to notice. Just before the family were about to disperse to their usual corners, Storm made her move.

"Peter, everyone, could you wait a minute?" She picked up her crutches and shot down the hall to her room, appearing seconds later with the bag. "Happy birthday, Peter. I know it's really tomorrow, but I just couldn't wait."

Her eyes shone with excitement, and Peter, who up until now had been somewhat unresponsive and tired, perked up with instant curiosity. He took the bag from Storm, gave her a kiss on the cheek, undid the ribbon, opened the bag and sat down on the chair as though someone had just removed his legs.

"Gosh!"

Every eye turned to Peter's face.

Storm laughed. "It's for your laptop, Peter, the one which goes faster."

"What's in the bag, Peter? Pair of old running shoes?" Ellen giggled at her own joke.

For answer Peter picked up the bag and emptied its contents on the table. There was a loud gasp from three dumbfounded spectators.

"How did you get all that?" Ellen exploded, jumping up from her chair. "Sell your body?"

"Ellen! Don't be crude," Basa scolded, staring at the pile in disbelief, too stunned to say anything else.

Andrew, turning towards the excited gift giver, spoke in a quiet voice. "Where did you get all this money, Storm?"

"I sold my paintings at the Village. When I'd sold them all, I bought some paper and drew people. They liked my drawings. I got twenty dollars each for them, that's the orange money, isn't it?"

There was stunned silence.

Basa recovered first. "Storm, dearest, did anyone ask your name?"

"Oh yes," Storm said. "There was the supermarket manager, his name's Matthew. He brings me lunch after I tripped up a villain who was in the car park, and he lets me use a big space in front of his shop. Then there's William who has the newsagency, that's where I get the paper, and today a funny man called Harry took pictures of me and told me I was a prodigy and going to be famous. He said he was from the voice, I didn't understand that bit."

"We're so screwed," Ellen exclaimed loudly.

"Ellen! That's enough." Basa glared at her daughter, but it was clear something had suddenly cast a different mood over the family gathering. Andrew was startled, Basa apprehensive, Ellen's eyes were brimming with what could have been excitement, and Peter was afraid. Afraid, yes, he was. Why? What was going on here?

"Have I done something wrong?" Storm's eyes were big and pleading.

"No, darling," Basa said, coming over and giving her a hug. "You've done something beautiful. It's just that there might be a problem—"

156

Basa turned sharply. Someone was knocking at the front door. Andrew glanced at his wife and headed down the hall.

A voice which Storm had heard before echoed from that direction. "Hi there. I'm Harry Sloane from the Northern Voice. May I come in? I believe this is where our Village artist lives? Won't keep you long, just wanted a name to put to the face."

"We're so screwed," Ellen muttered.

"Shut up Ellen." Peter glared at his sister. "Get this money off the table. Quick."

Three willing hands shovelled the whole lot back into the green bag. Basa took it into the kitchen and shoved it under the bench. Andrew and Harry Sloane emerged from the hallway.

"Ah, there she is," Harry beamed. "The child prodigy. I believe she could paint before she could talk, is that right?"

"Yes, that's right," Andrew said, real apprehension in his eyes.

Storm looked from face to face and wondered what had happened to her happy surprise.

"Now my dear," Sloane continued, "all I need is a name."

Everyone was staring at him as though he had grown another head. There was tension in the air. Silence. More silence. Still no one spoke.

"What's the matter?" Harry asked, perplexed. "All I want is a name. I know she calls herself Storm, but that's her artist's name. You can't mind me publishing her—"

"Ellen Craig."

All eyes turned towards Ellen who had spoken, her face flushed with an excited determination. "She's Ellen Craig," she went on. "This is Peter her brother."

"And you are?"

"Jasmine Delaney," Ellen smiled innocently at Sloane, "her cousin from Western Australia. I've come over for a long visit because my parents split up and—"

The expression on Basa's face was quite enough to silence further revelations. Storm was furious. She turned towards Ellen determined to correct her self-serving pretence, but Peter's hand suddenly squeezed her arm in a most meaningful way, and the look on his face didn't need any interpretation either. Harry smiled at the young girl and turned to face Andrew.

"Thanks for that. How long has she been crippled? Was it an accident? I guess she's finished school to concentrate on her art. Does she go to an Art College?"

"I do not give you permission to publish any other information about my daughter." Andrew said stiffly.

"Fair enough," Harry laughed. "The readers don't really want to know all that stuff anyway. I won't keep you anymore, Doctor Craig. Sorry for the interruption. Ciao!"

Andrew escorted Harry Sloane down the hall and out the front door.

Storm turned towards Ellen, furious. "Why you pretend?" she demanded. "Is this because of the tablecloth?"

"No," Ellen snapped, "it's to save you from your own stupidity."

"Ellen! For goodness sake," Basa groaned, very worried indeed. "Andrew, what do we do? It's only a matter of time."

"No it isn't," Ellen said confidently. "Nobody will ever check her age. Only slack reporters work for that rubbish. I throw it into the garbage every time it arrives on the front lawn."

STORM DANCING

Andrew frowned at his daughter, concern written deeply on his face. There was just a touch of admiration too. "I hope to goodness she's right," he heaved a sigh. "Perhaps it will only be a little picture buried amongst all the other rubbish nobody reads."

"What's happening? Why is everybody sad? What did I do?" Storm was practically in tears. Somehow Ellen had taken credit for all her artwork, Andrew and Basa were more worried than she had ever seen them, and Peter was afraid. This was certainly not the outcome she had intended.

Peter saw the tears forming in her eyes, came over and wrapped his arms around her, pushing her head into his shoulder.

"Storm, oh, Storm," he whispered softly into her ear, "I don't know how to say it properly. It's a... magnificent present, a stupendous present, the best I've ever had. I'll remember it all my life. You are so... so... beautiful, Storm. I love you."

He held her close rubbing his face in her hair. She had innocently put her life at risk, all for his sake. The more he thought about it the more choked up inside he became. He didn't want to let her out of his arms, she was safe there. Was she safe? He prayed Ellen's words would come true. Slowly he released her, and felt her hand come to rest within his own. She turned her face towards him, her lovely eyes filling with joy as she read the adoration in his. Basa, from the other side of the table, didn't miss that adoring expression either. Right now she had more pressing matters to attend to. She came around the table and squatted down beside Ellen so her face was on the same level as hers.

"Ellen that was very clever but very wrong. I know you did it for the best, thinking of Storm, but don't you see what trouble it will bring? What happens at school when your friends see the picture? When their mums see the picture?"

"You leave my friends to me," Ellen said with an air of confidence which made her mother even more anxious. "There'll be no problem from that direction."

Peter was still standing beside Storm holding her hand. He broke in to the conversation. "Storm doesn't know what's gone wrong. I think the first thing we should do is try to explain to her. How you explain to an angel what hell is like I don't know."

"You're right, Peter". Andrew came over to Storm and put his hands gently on her shoulders. His face was kind. "Young lady, you have made your family very proud of you today. We're all a bit stunned. I know Peter treasures your gift as he treasures you. That's not the problem at all."

"Why did Ellen say she was me?" Storm asked.

"Because Ellen has a name and you don't have one."

"But I'm Storm!"

"Yes, you are, bless you, but what's your other name, your family name?"

"Craig, like yours I suppose. I'm part of your family, aren't I?" Storm answered, tears welling up in her eyes.

Andrew put his arms around her and glanced helplessly towards Basa. He tried explain. "Of course you're part of our family. You will always be part of our family. You see, when Peter was born we had to fill in a paper with his name on it. That paper went to a place where they keep records of everyone who has been born in Australia. When Ellen was born we did the same thing. Their births are registered, that's what we call it."

"I'm not registered," Storm said, even more tearfully.

"Not as Storm Craig. If anyone were to check they would find out, and they would begin asking questions. They might want to know who you were and how you came here, and I couldn't tell them. Can you see what might happen?"

"Someone would come and take me away," Storm sobbed, tears streaming down her crumpled face.

"Not while I'm alive," Andrew said passionately. "Please don't cry, Storm. Oh dear, I've done it now."

Storm was clinging to him like the last tree trunk in a tidal wave, sobbing her heart out. The rest of the family gathered round them in a tight knot, which would have told any potential Storm remover they would have to remove the entire Craig family first. The feel of their arms enveloping her was somehow comforting, and after a while she stopped crying. Andrew picked her up in his arms and carried her onto the sofa. Basa sat down on the other side. Peter came over and stood nearby. Ellen sat on the carpet and curled herself round Storm's legs.

"I know," she said, "Peter could marry Storm and then she'd be a Craig. He's in love with her already."

Peter gave Ellen a look which would have wilted Hercules. He turned towards Storm, his face a bright red colour, hoping she hadn't heard. Her eyes told him she had.

"Peter's my brother," Storm said indignantly. "Of course he loves me. I love him too. That's silly talk. I do have a name, another name, don't I? Don't I?"

"Yes, Storm, you do, but I have no idea how we will ever find out what it was," Basa said in a worried voice.

"That was the me before me, wasn't it?"

"Yes darling."

"I don't want my before name," Storm said vehemently. "I want to be Craig, but I can't be. Is that right?"

"That's right," Basa said, apprehensively. "We may be able to do something called adopting you, making you officially our daughter, but I don't know how it would go. I think the fewer people who know about this the better. For the present you're Ellen Craig. Let's hope that holds water for a while. It was very clever of Ellen to think of that, even though it mightn't work. We'll have to see what's in the paper on Friday."

Peter went out of the room and returned with the green bag from the kitchen. He upended it on the floor and began to count out the notes.

"Is it enough?" Storm asked, the excitement returning to her voice. "If it isn't I'll draw some more".

"No you won't." Andrew attempted a laugh. "Not until this Ellen Craig stuff has died right down. How much is there, Peter?"

"Eighteen hundred and fifty dollars. Gosh!"

"Will it be enough?" Storm asked hopefully.

"Enough?" Peter shouted. "It'll buy the best laptop this family has ever seen!"

The evening ended on the happy note Storm had originally expected.

❋ ❋ ❋

Friday's edition of the Northern Voice was one which didn't end up in its usual place in the Craig's rubbish bin. Ellen bounded over the front lawn as soon as it landed, zipped it out of its plastic cover and opened the front page.

"We're so screwed," she muttered to herself and carried the paper back into the house.

Andrew had not gone into the surgery, and Basa had cancelled her first appointment. Peter was feeding crockery into the dishwasher and looking as apprehensive as he felt.

Ellen bounded into the room. "Front page spread," she announced loudly. "A huge picture. You can see right down Storm's boobs."

Andrew groaned and took the paper from his daughter's hand. Under the picture which Ellen had described so succinctly was a large headline:

STORM DANCING

PRODIGY ARTIST DRAWS CROWDS AT CHERRYBROOK VILLAGE

Miss Ellen Craig, who could draw before she could talk...

"We're so screwed."

"Ellen!" Basa barked loudly. "If I hear that revolting expression from your lips once more there will be no TV time this week!"

"Sorry Mum," Ellen said. "It's a pretty revealing picture of Storm, isn't it? If she wore her one piece costume she could charge people for taking her picture as well as for drawing theirs. She'd be even hotter in that."

"She will do no such thing," Basa said. "Where do you get all this nonsense from? I think we'll have to review the television programs you watch young lady."

Storm came into the room and Andrew handed her the paper.

"It's awful," she said, gawking at the picture. "Nobody will want to look at that. Right on top of the front page. I feel so... what's the word... embarrassed."

"For crying out loud," Ellen protested, "a lot of girls would kill to have boobs—"

"That's it, no screen time today," Basa snapped.

"Mum!"

"And it's time to get ready," Basa continued. "The school bus will be here in five minutes. I've got a job to go to, at least I did have before I got charged with falsifying evidence and people stealing."

"What's falsifying evidence and people stealing?" Storm asked anxiously.

"Never mind, Storm. Please stay inside today, and if anyone rings the doorbell let it ring. Don't answer it or the phone. You understand?"

"Yes, Mum."

"Andrew, will you keep an eye out for unwelcome strangers?"

"I'll brief Annette about the paper," Andrew nodded. "Have to tell her something."

"Tell her it's a misprint, of course," Ellen retorted in an exasperated tone.

"I'll think I'll start a new trend and tell her the truth. Get ready for school, Ellen. You'll miss the bus, and this is one morning I don't want to drive you."

※ ※ ※

Ellen didn't miss the bus. She arrived at school, stowed her bag in her locker down the hall and went into her classroom, noticing several girls tittering to themselves as she passed. The teacher was late. Samantha Higgins, who Ellen hated with a passion, fired the first salvo.

"We didn't know you'd grown such big knockers, Ellen. Where do you hide them?"

Ellen resisted the temptation to discolour the floor with the remains of Samantha's face, and replied in a voice loud enough for every girl in the room to hear. "It's a misprint, you dork. Should read Helen Craig, my dad's brother's daughter. She's staying with us. Her parents had to go to Afghanistan in a hurry because they're working with the United Nations. You know that bloody paper never gets it right."

The swear word was a late edition to the story Ellen had been constructing in her head since the previous evening. Swear words were always needed with girls like Samantha Higgins, they just didn't understand a sentence without them. The teacher came into the room then, but from the way Samantha and several other girls seemed to lose immediate interest, she knew the ploy had worked. She glanced at her good friend Tamsin Lucas and knew it hadn't. More work was needed. Her fertile little mind went into overdrive until the bell sounded for morning recess. Pushing her way over to Tamsin, she grabbed her arm and piloted her out of the room down the corridor, a conspiratorial expression on her face. Towards the end of the building there was an empty classroom with an open door. Ellen shoved her friend inside and shut it behind her.

"What are we doing here?" Tamsin said, more than a little annoyed at being pushed around. "And why did you give out all that rubbish about the girl being your cousin? Your dad's brother doesn't have a daughter. I know, my dad works with him on the police force. He's not married."

"Keep your voice down." Ellen crouched under one of the desks and pulled her friend close beside her, whispering loudly in her ear. "If someone heard what you were saying Manon Desalle could be murdered. Chopped up while she was still alive."

The other girl stared at Ellen in alarm. "Who's this Manon person?"

"The girl in the photograph, stupid. She's in the Witness Protection program. Interpol have hidden her in our home. She's the only living witness to a horrible serial killer. The other victims were chopped to pieces – while they were still alive, one after the other."

Tamsin thought she was going to be sick.

Ellen went on, her voice edged with excitement. "You see the murderer only knows her name, he doesn't know what she looks like. If the paper printed her real name he'd come and drag her away to some quarry to chop her up – with an axe. The police have been after him for months. Swear you'll say nothing. I've only told you because you're my best friend."

Tamsin had always suspected that being Ellen's best friend would one day present difficulties, but never this sort. She didn't quite believe her, but then she didn't quite disbelieve her either. In any case it was such an exciting, scary secret, worth knowing at any price.

"I swear I'll never say a thing," she said breathlessly. "Do we spit on each other's hands now, or something? Do we make a blood oath of silence? I have a pin from my badge here. We could prick our fingers and—"

"Your word is enough for me, Tamsin," Ellen said hastily. "Friends trust one another. Remember, not one word, even to your parents, even the other girls in our group, okay?"

"I swear. There's the bell. Do you want some fruitcake? I don't like it."

"Later, come on."

Ellen came back to her seat in the classroom fairly confident her schemes had worked out. The girls would tell their mothers it was a misprint if they asked, and Tamsin would shut up about the whole thing. She turned her attention to the teacher who had just come into the room.

❋ ❋ ❋

James Hunt stared at the picture on the front page of the Northern Voice for quite a long time before replacing it carefully on top of his desk. So Sloane had beaten him to the front page again, and looking at the photo he could tell why. He recognised the girl from the lemonade stand. Ellen Craig, eh? Who called herself Storm. The other girl had said her name was Stornway. He had thought it odd at the time. Logging on to his computer he typed a few keys then sat back thoughtfully in his chair. Ellen Craig, only daughter of Drs. Andrew and Basa Craig, was all of eleven years eight months old. How curious.

He called to Sloane who occupied the cubical on the other side of the divider. "Sloane, how did you get the name of that young artist? Did she tell you herself?"

Sloane shuffled a few papers on his desk, stood up and came over into Hunt's cubicle. "No, the girl kept giving me her artist's name, Storm. Suppose she didn't trust a stranger. Don't blame her really. You never know these days," he grunted.

"Anyway, I found out where she lived and got the name from her family. They have another girl living with them, a Jasmine Delaney – parents from Western Australia, split up. She was the first person to volunteer Ellen's name. Some reticence about having his daughter on the front page. Don't know why. Anyway, her father, Dr. Andrew Craig confirmed it. Why are you interested? The story's mine, mate, and if there's any follow up I'm going to do it."

"No follow up. Was the Jasmine girl short with blonde hair and blue eyes?"

"Yeah. You've met her?"

"Probably not. Thanks, Sloane."

"She's pretty hot, that Storm girl."

"Yeah, I saw the picture."

"Look better in a bikini. Look even better under the shower wearing raindrops."

"Yeah. Thanks, Sloane. Sorry to disturb you."

Sloane went back into his cubicle. Hunt navigated away from the web page he had been browsing and cleared the computers browsing history. So Ellen Craig was calling herself Jasmine Delaney, and the Storm girl was calling herself Ellen Craig, and the good Dr. Craig was verifying the whole pack of lies. How interesting, how very interesting. Of course Sloane would want to see her naked, he never thought above his crotch at the best of times.

Naked... and suddenly an extraordinary thought. He knew exactly how she would look in Sloane's preferred manner of dress, exactly because he had seen her wearing it. The room had been dark, and there was a lot of company. He remembered being bored and half plastered, or was it half bored and totally plastered? Besides, it was years ago. Perhaps it was just his repressed sexual fantasy playing games with his mind. Nonetheless there were strange doings afoot and he was going to get to the bottom of them.

CHAPTER 15

Detective Inspector Ray Wright sat forward in his chair, and watched the steady crawl of commuter traffic on Ryde Road several floors below him, almost grateful for the mountain of work which prevented him joining it. Pulling a thick folder from a filing cabinet at arm's reach, he placed it on his desk, leant over to the intercom and spoke to his secretary.

"Send Brian Craig in, would you, Janice?" He opened the folder and studied the picture which he had stuck on the front page. She was certainly a pretty girl, no doubt about it.

There was a knock at the door, and Sergeant Brian Craig stepped into the room. "You called, boss?"

"I did," Wright said. "Have you read the latest edition of the Craig Family News?" He tossed a sheaf of papers towards Brian, who had seated himself on the only other chair in the room.

"I have. Pretty comprehensive, aren't they? Andrew told you he'd keep you informed."

"Superfluous citizens interest me, Craig, especially when they're about eighteen years old – or look it," Wright continued, touching his fingers together. "I think to myself, where did they spend the last seventeen years? What were they doing? And in this case, what happened to the girl's memory? Are we dealing with a massive case of medical malpractice, or a possible felon with extraordinary theatrical skills?"

"You know she's no felon," Brian said defensively. "By now you will have made a very thorough check with Interpol and our American friends. Nothing came up, did it?"

"You know me well, Craig," Wright smiled slightly. "You can tell that to the good doctor Craig if you wish. He's certainly kept his side of the bargain." He shuffled through the large file and eventually withdrew a single sheet of paper. "That isn't why I called you in here. Someone else is taking an interest in our superfluous citizen."

"Who might that be?" Brian raised his eyebrows.

"A reporter by the name of James Hunt, works for some local rag called the Northern Voice." Wright tossed the front page of the paper towards Brian. "Turned up at Hornsby Police Station the other day with that picture of the girl, wanting to know if she was on a missing persons list. The officer apparently asked why she would be missing when her name was Ellen Craig, so what was he getting at? The guy was persistent enough to raise the constable's attention. After he'd gone, the officer checked Ellen Craig's age. Then he checked the missing persons. Finally he identified the girl from the file we sent around after the storm, and rang me."

"And you told him what?" Brian frowned heavily.

"That we were keeping an eye on the situation, and would he let us know if Hunt turned up again, or anyone else." He shuffled the pictures back into the file. "He said he would. I asked him to keep the matter between ourselves for the time being."

"Thanks."

"It wasn't out of consideration for you," Wright said levelly. "I want to find out who this girl is, Craig. People don't just appear on the planet unless they're aliens, and for my money that girl seems very human to me."

"Do I tell the Craigs?" Brian asked in the same level voice.

"No need to alarm them. I think we'll play our own game for a while."

"Know why she was selling her art in the Village?" Brian grinned, "She wanted to buy my nephew a laptop when his old one broke. She's a real darling," he added. "You should come around and talk to her."

Wright nodded slightly. "That's all, Craig. This is between ourselves for the time being. There's something here that doesn't smell right, and I'm going to find out what it is, darling or no darling."

Brian left the room, his face beginning to betray his worried thoughts. There was a man who had come up to the girls when they were running a lemonade stall at the local garage and asked some questions. Perhaps this was the same man. Perhaps he had checked Ellen's age for himself and was simply curious. Perhaps there was a lot more to it. He would spend the next hour making sure he knew everything there was to know about James Hunt. In the meantime, blood was thicker than water. He picked up the phone and dialled Andrew.

Chapter 16

Rachel Demarra put down her glass of champagne and stared out the window of her very comfortable apartment on the seventh floor South LaBrea Avenue, Hollywood. Outside it was hot and uncomfortable, inside it was cool and pleasant. The air conditioner hummed softly in the background, Chopin was playing on the stereo. Alan was in the bathroom enjoying a shower after the evening's bedroom gymnastics. Roger had oozed off into the sunset the day after the compensation payment had come through. How different was life now. She remembered the day she had arrived at the small downtown pad Roger had promised to set up for them, only to find another woman had already taken up residence in the few weeks before her arrival.

Roger had explained that until he had heard of Felicity's tragic death he had expected Rachel to stay in Australia, and, well, man was not made to live alone. Rachel had removed the usurper by the simple expedient of bundling all her clothes into a bag and dumping them in the trash can on the pavement outside the hotel. Lucy had come home tired and in need of love that evening, only to discover some homeless person reefing through her underwear. There had been a very intense scene in the apartment afterwards. Roger had played the role of the gutless bastard, Rachel the jealous lover successfully executing her revenge, and Lucy the jilted and furious tart who was about to get her comeuppance in the hands of a much more experienced player. Their relationship had begun to sour from that point on, to the day when Rachel had written him a note, telling him she had moved to a decent apartment for a change and would he, Roger, keep it that way by getting to blazes out of her life.

She would have been surprised to learn how relieved he felt.

Her first film, A Severe Justice, had done well in Cannes, and whilst not being a box office wonder, had turned in a healthy profit. She had played the part of Dr. Sally Jacobsen, an industrial chemist, horribly disfigured in an accident for which she was not responsible, fighting for the compensation she deserved. The plot bore a faint resemblance to the drama happening in her own life, especially the compensation bit, and she had turned out a pretty good performance, not Oscar class, but good enough for her to get another part weeks after the first screening.

Her next picture was an animated feature called Kalia Jan, in which she was the voice of the central character, a princess of the same name. This had gone really well. International release following on weeks after the premiere performance in the States. Four months later it still had not gone to DVD. Pity no one saw her on the screen, but her reputation as an actress was slowly but surely climbing. She had already been approached by a couple of directors, one of whom wanted to shoot in Australia. She had turned him down straight away. Australia was still too close, too painful.

She stroked the lucky black stone on the coffee table with her foot. Yes, she could still feel its soothing power. This was a good apartment, its Feng Shui a perfect balance, number 77 on the 7th floor. The stone was the same one her therapist in Australia had given her, and she had acquired several other potent charms since her stay in LA had begun. A red rock from Sedona which harnessed Vortex energy, a lucky crystal she had picked up somewhere in Yavapai country, a Navaho talisman of great power she had bought at a roadside stall. Yes, all these were exerting a calming, empowering influence on her life. She had met Alan on the third of March while sitting at Delphine's Bistro, table number three. The rest was a foregone conclusion. He had turned out to be a lover who put Roger to shame in every department.

She thought back to those last horrible days in Australia. Yet it could have been worse, if Felicity had returned to consciousness and invaded her world like a deadly virus. All her artistic soul would have been sucked out of her, poisoning her every breath. Life would have turned into hell itself. How she had suffered in those last agonising days. An artist, she reflected, had to suffer to become an artist. This was the path she had chosen for herself, and so the suffering had to come, refining, building, teaching her how to feel deep empathy for the characters she portrayed. Now she had become a name for herself, Rachel hoped very much that no more suffering would be required.

CHAPTER 17

"Y ou're not going there, and that's final," Andrew said firmly.

Storm turned her big brown eyes up into his face with a sorrowful expression, carefully calculated to produce sufficient deep regret in his heart to make him change his mind.

"And it's no use using those eyes on me either," Andrew said, trying hard to maintain his serious expression. "You've been learning from Ellen. Second thoughts, perhaps she's been taking lessons from you."

Storm dissolved into laughter which totally spoiled the effect. "I know you're right, Daddy, but Matthew will be sorry," she said. "I think a lot of people went into his shop after they bought a picture."

"I'll ring him and tell him you didn't want all the publicity. I'll say you'll be back when it's died down a bit," Andrew assured her.

"Thanks."

"Next time you go I'm coming with you," Peter interrupted with a determined expression that Storm didn't even try to dislodge. She could see her Village visits would be postponed for quite some time.

Peter's exams were in a few weeks now, and she knew how important they were for him. He would repeat the year, he said, if he didn't get the marks for Medicine, and she didn't want him to. The laptop had been bought and Peter was delighted with it. He had shown Storm all the things it could do, and the girl had drawn more from his delight than the confusing array of images which had flashed before her eyes. She gave Peter one of her and-I-love-you-too smiles and walked slowly towards the lounge room where Ellen was watching TV.

"Do you have anything else I could read?" she asked.

"Not now, Storm," Ellen said crossly. "Can't you see I'm busy? We have to go and see that movie, Kalia Jan. Everyone is saying it's great."

"What are you talking about?"

"Check out my room. All my books are in there," Ellen said, her face still glued to the screen.

"Thanks."

Storm didn't feel too thankful. There was a desk with bookshelves in Ellen's room, but they contained anything but books. Ellen's book filing system was a pile of chaos on the floor. If you wanted one you rummaged the pile. Somehow the girl seemed to know just how deep to dig when she wanted anything, but Storm knew she didn't have the knack at all. Several times she had sorted Ellen's books out and placed them carefully on the shelves. They had gradually ended up on the floor again as more important items took their place. She glanced at the pile and groaned softly. One book remained on the shelves, a rather fat one. Ellen had never recommended it, and she had never thought to read it because of its size. Large books usually meant lots of large words and long sentences, and Storm found them tiring. Basa had a lot of books about medical things which fitted into this category, but Storm loved the pictures. The human body was so beautifully designed, so perfectly put together. Why had someone attached such big complicated words to the various structures in it? Peter's books were much the same without the fascinating pictures.

She took the book from the shelf and read the cover. Children's Bible. *Wonder what that is?* Storm thought to herself. *Let's see if its readable.* She turned the first page, and to her delight found that she could understand every word. *Good enough for me,* she thought, and tucking the book under her arm she walked slowly to her own bedroom where the sound of the television blasting out its discordant message was faint enough to be ignored. It took so long to walk without crutches, but Andrew and Basa had insisted she do it for at least half an hour every day, and she had been faithful to their wishes. Each step was an effort of concentration, and as soon as she didn't watch what her right foot was doing she fell over. Certain parts of her anatomy had developed a fierce dislike of falling over. It was so much easier on crutches. Storm closed her bedroom door, curled herself up on her bed and opened the book.

Two hours later Andrew popped in to tell her dinner was ready. "What's that you're reading, Storm?" he asked.

"Children's Bible," Storm said enthusiastically. "It's a good story. Coming, Dad."

After dinner and stacking the dishwasher, she went back and kept reading.

Ellen was the next interruption. "You want to come and play Blokus?" Storm loved Blokus.

"No thanks Ellen. I'm caught up in a book."

"What book?"

"Children's Bible."

"That rubbish," Ellen snorted. "I'll play with mum."

It was late that night before Storm went to sleep. This book was different. It said it was about things which had actually happened, and not some made up fairy tale. She liked the way the characters were real, although the things they did quite shocked her sometimes. It talked about God too, the person Andrew had mentioned once before. He was awesome, too big to imagine, but He fascinated her. She thought about the world around her, its intricate beauty, the vastness of the stars in the night sky. So all this was created by God. It made perfect sense.

The next day was Saturday. Storm liked Saturdays because Andrew and Basa were at home for most of the time. Breakfast was later and everything was more relaxed, except for Peter who hardly emerged from his bedroom these days. Andrew came into the breakfast room carrying two empty teacups, which meant he was ready for breakfast, and Basa would soon emerge clad in a dressing gown. Andrew always seemed content in some way when he brought those cups back. He smiled at Storm, engrossed in her book at the kitchen table. Ellen was still in bed and the TV was silent.

"Morning Storm," he greeted her with a kiss on her cheek. "Still reading your Children's Bible?"

Storm gave him a beautiful good-morning smile. "Love the hero."

"Have you been reading all night?"

"No, got up early." She closed the book and gave him one of her irresistible smiles. "Dad, would you do something for me?"

"How can I refuse when you look at me that way?"

Storm laughed. "I got all that money but I couldn't count it. I didn't know how to do the... sums? Is that the right word, sums?"

"Uh huh."

"Could you teach me how to do sums? If you have time. I'd ask Peter but I know he hasn't."

"No problem," Andrew said, placing the cups on the kitchen sink. "How about after breakfast? I'm starving."

So began Storm's home schooling. Andrew found she was good at picking up mathematical ideas, and Basa, not wishing to be left out of the program, said she would teach her some simple biology. Ellen said she couldn't imagine why anyone would want to learn biology. She was going to be a lawyer and make squillions of dollars. Medicine was boring and doctors worked far too hard.

So over the next couple of weeks Andrew taught her maths, Basa taught her biology, and Ellen taught her patience, because she was finding it hard to cope with the transformation in her former baby sister. Storm seemed to have suddenly grown wiser. Even though she could never match Ellen's extraordinary skill with words, her speech had developed a certain graciousness, a deeper understanding which Ellen grudgingly recognised but would never acknowledge. Something in Storm had changed since she read that stupid Children's Bible, but Ellen had poured so much scorn on her for doing it, that her pride prevented her from asking Storm what it was and how it had happened.

Then there was the unfortunate incident with the CD. Ellen had been given a free CD of songs when she walked out of school one day. She had taken them home, played one, discovered it was all about that Bible stuff and chucked the CD into her pile on the floor of the family room. *Should have been the rubbish bin,* Ellen thought unhappily. *Now see what's happened. I suppose it's her childish mind which makes her go for all that.*

Not only had Storm found the CD and played it, she spent an infuriatingly large part of the day singing the blasted songs herself.

> "Jesus is the boss
> Jesus is the boss
> Jesus is the boss
> Of me!"

Over and over again. It wasn't the quality of her voice, it was the volume. Now her stupid brother was sometimes joining in. Of course he was, he was besotted with the girl, anyone could see that. She was draining his brain. By the time he got to university he would fail everything, because he was already acting stupid.

The night before Peter's first exam in English finally arrived. The family had an early tea, and after dessert Basa brought out a bottle of sparkling apple juice and poured a glass for everyone.

"To Peter," she said, "for results which do justice to his hard faithful study."

"To Peter," Ellen said, "becoming a lawyer instead."

Storm frowned. "Why do we do this?"

"Tradition," Andrew said. "It's supposed to bring good luck."

"What's luck?" Storm raised a questioning eyebrow.

"Good luck is when everything just happens to work out right," Basa said, smiling.

"Oh. For no reason then."

Andrew laughed. "It's just another way of telling Peter we all hope the exam goes really well and we care about him."

There was a curious expression on Storm's face. Peter went back into his room for a final squiz over his English notes, and an hour or so later he heard a soft knock at the door.

"Can the distraction come in for just a moment?"

"Come in, Storm."

Storm came in, and in her usual fashion made herself comfortable on the bed. Peter came over and sat on the edge, wondering what had occasioned this evening's visit.

"Peter," Storm said seriously, "you can't add a single hour to your life by worrying about it. When you follow Jesus he'll take care of you. Don't worry about tomorrow, Peter, let it worry about itself. Each day has enough trouble of its own."

Peter turned round and stared at her. "Where did you get this from?"

"Children's Bible."

"Storm, I don't want you to end up disillusioned with this following Jesus stuff."

Storm smiled at him. "You think it's like following Peter Pan or someone like Mother Theresa, don't you, but it's not. One isn't real and the other's dead. Jesus is real and he's alive."

"You actually believe that?" Peter said, wrinkling his forehead.

"Of course, Peter. Everyone else has wished you this luck, but I don't understand about luck. Can I pray for you?"

"What?" Peter asked, seriously surprised.

She uncurled herself and sat up beside him, putting her arm around his shoulder.

"Jesus, please help Peter not to worry about his English exam tomorrow, because he is, even though he's pretending he's not."

She reached over and kissed him on the cheek, smiled and stood up ready to leave.

"That's it?" Peter asked incredulous.

"That's it," Storm laughed. "You don't need heaps of words. Goodnight Peter."

With that she walked very slowly and carefully out of the room, leaving a rather stunned Peter behind her. It wasn't so much what she had done, it was the unnerving certainty in the way she had done it. Surely this was simply another expression of Storm's delightful childlikeness that she would accept what she had read. Yet there was a quality in her naïve trust which defied description, a quality which was somehow compelling of belief. Peter stripped off his clothes, got into his pyjamas and into bed. Thinking about Storm rather than worrying about his English paper, he was asleep in all of five minutes.

CHAPTER 18

Frankfurt that same year

G rüße Tante Frieda" Gerhardt Metzger took his aunt's hand and raised it to his lips in an old fashioned gesture of respect. "Sie suchen seit Ihrer Rückkehr aus dem Krankenhaus gesund."[1]

The old lady beckoned him to an armchair in front of the fire. The winter in Frankfurt had been severe that year. Snow lay thick on the ground, and a bitter wind still blew far too often for comfort. Her nephew sank wearily into the comfortable leather, and slowly shuffling a short distance, she seated herself on the tall spindle backed chair on the other side of the fireplace. It wasn't as comfortable, but it was firmer and higher and easier to get out of. She composed her unsteady hands in her lap and replied, a trace of sadness in her voice.

"The cancer is aggressive and inoperable, Gerhardt. It was a most unexpected diagnosis. I'm sure you know that, so stop trying to patronise me. I have a year, perhaps less than a year."

"Yes, I learned that from Johann at the clinic. I'm sorry, Tante Frieda. It is the way of life, is it not, birth then death. Nothing can prevent it yet. One day maybe, but then it is perhaps a foolish thing to seek to live forever."

---

[1] You are looking well since your return from hospital

"On the Earth, yes. But we will live forever in heaven."

"I'm glad you find such belief a comfort, Tante. Myself, I take comfort in reality not fairy tales, but I'm glad they bring you peace."

"Ah, Gerhardt, you are far too much the rationalist. You have such a mechanical perspective on life. We are all machines, are we not? You have never married, Gerhardt. Perhaps this is why. Machines cannot love or give love. Surely loneliness is not to be rejoiced in?"

"I am more than content with my work, Tante. Shall we talk about something else?"

Tante Frieda sighed. There was a certain coldness in her nephew which disturbed her, even frightened her sometimes. She remembered the young boy who delighted to accompany her to the Lutherischen Kirche not far from where she once lived. Then his parents had become divorced, and he had changed. The long years of her daughter's bitterness had soaked into his own soul, yes, and he had taken refuge in his work, allowed it to consume him to the exclusion of all else. First a medical doctor, then a doctorate in neurophysiology followed by a lectureship at Goethe-Universität, finally a professorship. At what cost, she thought to herself. She changed the subject.

"I had a phone call from Gladys Machen yesterday, you remember, my friend who went on that Australian tour with me a couple of months ago. She is well and planning another trip to Canada. She asked me if I would like to go... I said I would... but I will not."

"I'm truly glad you managed to see at least some of the world before you became unwell, Tante. Australia is a remarkable country, so diverse, so much empty space."

"Yes. The portrait came from there. A young girl, very talented."

She pointed to the drawing enclosed in a wooden frame hanging on the wall opposite the fire.

"She was indeed," Metzger agreed. "I suppose you paid a great many euros for it, Tante."

"Not at all, only twenty Australian dollars. I'm not sure how many euros that comes to. She did it in a few minutes while I sat on a chair. That sheet of paper was on the ground, and she only glanced up at me a few times. The girl must have had a photographic memory. You were in Australia just over a year ago, were you not, Gerhardt? Then you returned as suddenly as you went. Even your own mother did not realise you had gone, and none of us expected your return. You must learn to communicate more with those who love you, Gerhardt."

"Indeed I must, Tante," Metzger sighed. "It was a split second decision because Isaac invited me to do some interesting research with him. He was very excited and would not hear of a delay. The research project ended, and I came home. One day I would like to carry on with that research if I ever had opportunity to do so."

"You were great friends, you and Isaac, in your undergraduate days at the medizinische Fakultät. Yet now, when I ask you how he is you cannot answer me. Is he still in Australia?"

"No, he is at MIT in America. They were glad to have him back I believe. It's true, Tante, we were estranged towards the end of the project. Isaac became inconsistent, sentimental, irrational. We argued. I will not work with him again, or if I do it will be on a project that I am in charge of. He's a brilliant man. I was sorry he allowed his feelings to overpower his rationality."

"Ah, there is hope for him. His grandparents suffered so terribly. Such a gentle boy. I am sorry to hear your long friendship has come to an end. Perhaps he has discovered some truths you need to learn, Gerhardt."

"I think not, Tante Frieda. Now I must be going. I have a lecture in less than an hour. I will call in again next week. Remember, whenever you would like to end the pain, I can assist you."

"No, Gerhardt," Tante Frieda protested gently. "I will allow God to take me home in his time, not yours. I pray for you, Gerhardt, you are a man without love, and a man without purpose."

Professor Gerhardt Metzger got up from the armchair, came over to his aunt and kissed her hand. "Do not get up, Tante, I will see myself out. I may be a man without love, but not without purpose. Until next week."

He walked over to the stand near the hall, pulled his greatcoat off the rack and put it on. A red and black woollen scarf came after that, and a black woollen cap the finishing touch. With a final wave of his hand he went down the hall, opened the front door and stepped out into the bitter wind. She would not last the next twelve months. Home care would eventually become a necessity, then home nursing. In the end she would return to the hospital to die. He could have made dying so much easier for her if she had agreed. A nice cup of tea, a gentle prick in the arm, and a painless sleep accompanied by the music of her beloved Johann Sebastian Bach. But no, the same irrational stupidity prevented it, the constricting belief in some metaphysical universe. There was some God to whom she was responsible, to whose heavenly bliss she would be welcomed when finally the dark finality of death would painfully overtake her. At least Isaac was right in that. So much blood and pain had been caused by religion. It took him several attempts to start his car. With the engine running, he turned up the heat to full blast and headed off towards the university for his neurology lecture.

CHAPTER 19

Peter had finished his exams with a great deal more confidence than he had begun. He had done well, he knew, but had he done well enough? Now it was a waiting game, and it didn't pay to think about it too much. Andrew and Basa were incredibly encouraging. Ellen who was due to turn twelve in a few weeks, kept trying to persuade him to do anything else rather than sell himself into medical slavery for the rest of his life. Storm assumed an air of quiet but unshakeable confidence, which Peter found encouraging and disturbing at the same time. Following his exams he had gone out with friends on a few occasions, but now spent most of his time around the house, and most of that taking over Storm's mathematical education. Her skill in maths had grown to the point where Peter felt she could pass some of his year eleven assignments. Finally he gave her one, and was overjoyed when she scored eleven out of a possible twenty. Storm was bitterly disappointed. She virtually dragooned Peter into teaching her for three hours every morning after breakfast, and a couple of weeks later demanded another assignment.

"Don't you dare make it easier," she warned. "I can tell if you do, and I will be very cross."

Peter had made it harder and she had scored nineteen out of twenty, which made Storm very happy and Peter very relieved. Basa had switched from Biology to English, because she was finding some concepts difficult to explain, and Andrew switched to simple chemistry. They tried to spend an hour every couple of days teaching her, but work often interfered. Only Ellen regarded the studious atmosphere in her home with a jaundiced eye. Sometimes a family could become so boring.

It was then they simultaneously made a startling and mostly welcome discovery. Basa had given Storm a copy of Great Expectations by Charles Dickens, because that was one of the set Higher School Certificate texts last year. Storm became engrossed in it, finished it in all of two days, and left it lying on the breakfast table.

Ellen picked it up over breakfast, opened it to page one and cast a disparaging eye over the contents. "You couldn't read this in two days," she said with absolute certainty. "Bet you skimmed it."

"No, I read it," Storm objected. "Mr. Dickens has such a beautiful way with words."

"Don't believe you," Ellen replied defensively.

Storm shut her eyes for a second, opened them and began. "As I never saw my father or my mother, err... and never saw any likeness of either of them ... for their days were long before the days of photographs, my first fancies regarding what they were like, were unreasonably derived from their tombstones. The shape of the letters on my father's, gave me an odd idea that he was a square, stout, dark man, with curly black—"

Ellen dropped the book onto the table and stared at Storm with her mouth open.

Basa, coming in from the kitchen, stopped suddenly. "What was that you said, Storm?" she asked.

"From the character and turn of the inscription... 'Also Georgiana Wife of the above,' I drew a childish conclusion that my mother was freckled and sickly.' I think that's how it goes. I remember the first page very clearly. I think Mr. Dickens must have taken a lot of trouble with that first page. Why is everyone staring at me?"

"She's got a bloody photographic memory!" Ellen exclaimed bitterly. "Life just isn't fair."

"Ellen! How many times do I have to warn you about language?" Basa said sharply. Then in an inquiring tone, "err... Storm, how much more can you remember like that?"

It turned out Storm could only remember a few paragraphs word perfect from her reading, but when she scanned a page briefly she could read it back from memory while someone else held the book to check. Ellen, the would-be lawyer, went straight into a decline. The rest of the family were jumping around in excitement.

"You're brilliant," Peter said excitedly, putting Mr. Dickens back down on the table after the latest demonstration. "You'll ace any English exam. When did you know you could do that, Storm?"

"I didn't think it was special," Storm replied, a small frown crossing her face. "That's how I draw things. I remember what they look like. It's really nothing."

"It really isn't nothing," Andrew said, shaking his head slightly. "I think our Storm is going to add to the Craig family's reputation for academic excellence."

"What *would* you like to study, Storm?" Peter asked.

"Art, stupid. What else?" Ellen was feeling very put out.

"No. Why should I?" Storm said, surprised. "I can draw already. No, I want to be a doctor."

Stunned silence followed that innocent announcement.

Basa recovered first. She came over to Storm and hugged her. "That's a wonderful idea. This family will do everything we can to get you there."

Andrew was still getting over the shock. Visions of Storm standing naked in the kitchen, pouring milk all over herself nearly twelve months ago, came back into his mind. The child they had once thought belonged in a sheltered workshop, a psychiatric centre for the intellectually disabled, wanted to become a doctor. It was an overwhelming thought. Whether Basa felt the same he didn't know, but the expression on her face was suggestive of the same surprise.

Then and there the Craig family made a plan for Storm's education. She would be home schooled for one more year then attend a college of Technical and Further Education. She would sit for her HSC the year after next. Andrew had a patient who had done that, and found it a better learning environment than returning to school. The year's home schooling would give Storm a head start in Maths, English, History and probably Biology as well, if Basa and Andrew could overcome the practical work problem. All Storm would have to do to be in the running was to pick up Chemistry, and Peter could give her some background in that as well.

After all the excitement died down, Peter helped her walk out into the back yard and sat down on the swing seat with her.

"It's very hard to get the marks you need, Storm," he said in a worried voice. "I don't want you to study so hard that something … happens to you." He stared steadily at the ground near his feet. "I would much rather you be an artist and be like you are than … than…"

"Turn into what I was before I came here?" Storm reached for his hand.

"Yeah."

"Do you know what I think happened to me?" Storm squeezed his hand, and watched him turn his troubled eyes towards her.

"No. What?"

"Come closer, put your hands on my head and part my hair around the back." She moved her head forward and down so he could. "No, down a bit more, there. See?"

"What are they?" Peter asked, alarmed.

"Cranial surgery. Surgeries. I've had lots. Someone spent a long time opening my head and doing things to my brain."

Peter was stunned. He lifted Storm's hair around the side of her head following the marks, all of them in parallel. Finally he lifted her head up gently until her lovely eyes were filling his sight.

"Has Dad or Mum seen these?" he asked gently.

"They saw them the day I came here. I discovered them a few months ago while I was brushing my hair. I'm growing it longer and straighter, you see. I've talked to Mum about it. She told me what it might mean. She was really upset that I'd found them."

"Someone damaged your brain deliberately?" Peter asked, aghast.

"It seems to work alright though, doesn't it?" She took hold of his hands in her own and held them together in her lap. "Except for the walking. That bit doesn't, and I don't think it ever will, not properly." She squeezed his hands together in her own. "I don't know what happened, but every time I think about it, this terrible fear comes all over me. Not like it did at first, before you all came to love me. I talk to Jesus about it now."

She gripped his hands tightly. "I go cold all of a sudden. I tried to draw it, the fear shape. God pulled me away from it, Peter, but it's still there somewhere, waiting. When I think about it coming for me I have to pray very hard."

Peter met her frightened eyes with his own. "I want to pray with you," he said quietly.

On December the eighteenth someone from the Board of Studies rang to say Peter had come eleventh in the State. The entire Craig household went into rapture. Andrew took them all out to the Benelong restaurant at the Opera House that evening for a celebratory meal. Storm had a glass of wine, enjoyed it very much, and fell asleep before dessert with her head on Peter's shoulder. Ellen ate Storm's strawberry Pavlova with blueberries and cream as well as her own, keeping a watchful eye on the girl's state of consciousness while she did. Peter wrapped his left arm around her so she wouldn't fall off his shoulder. Certain male patrons on other tables were staring in his direction with envy in their eyes. Peter knew that look. There was no way he was going to tell them the girl snuggling in his neck thought of him as her brother. In some ways he wished she didn't.

The euphoria in the Craig household lasted for most of the following week. There were meetings Peter had to go to, a photo shoot with the Northern Voice, and a radio interview with some of the other candidates who had done well.

❋ ❋ ❋

Storm decided to return to the Village on Saturdays to draw people, because she wanted to buy the family some Christmas presents. Peter decided to go with her. On the first Saturday Storm didn't earn a cent, but the Craig family acquired a new pet.

Storm went straight into the supermarket to say "hello" to Matthew, only to hear his agitated voice coming from the refrigerated goods section. She decided to investigate. Matthew's right hand was wrapped in a bloodstained handkerchief.

"What happened?" Storm came towards him on her crutches. "Matthew, you've hurt your hand."

"Hurt my hand?" Matthew muttered angrily. "That flea-bitten fur bag over there is the thing that's hurt my hand." He grinned sheepishly, "Hello, Storm, great to have you back."

Storm turned her head towards the refrigerator. There in the corner was a large black Persian cat, its front paw defensively extended. In its mouth was a sausage, part of a long string of them which the animal had grabbed from the refrigerator. Storm laughed out loud.

"It's not a laughing matter," Matthew said, looking wounded. "That brute should be put down. This isn't the first time she's helped herself to my sausages. Don't get near her whatever you do. She's pretty handy with her claws."

"Peter, take these will you?" Storm said, handing her crutches over to him.

"I really don't think you should get any closer, Storm," Peter warned. "If she scratches you I'll have to take you home straight away for a tetanus shot."

Undeterred, Storm made her way slowly and awkwardly towards the animal. When she was close enough, she dropped to her knees, reached out and began to stroke the cat behind the ears. She dropped the sausages and pushed her head against Storm's hand, obviously appreciating the treatment. Matthew and Peter watched anxiously.

"Anytime now she's going to get it," Matthew muttered. "Oh goodness, she's picked the animal up!"

Peter watched fascinated as Storm cuddled the cat into her arms, talking softly and stroking it all the time.

"She's so beautiful," Storm laughed softly. "Come on Peter, let's take her home. I've always wanted a cat. Do you want to hold her?"

Peter declined. Holding Storm's crutches, and doing his best to support her on his arm without annoying the cat, they made their long, slow way back to the car. By the time they reached it the cat was lying on its back in Storm's arms, purring loudly. Peter shook his head. *She has an incredible way with animals,* he thought. *If I'd picked up that fleabag I would have needed medical attention.*

"I hope Mum and Dad don't mind," Storm said with a worried face. "I'd hate to have to take her back. She's so nice. See? She just loves me stroking her tummy."

Peter opened the car door, and helped Storm into the front seat, cat and all. "I think you're fairly safe," he laughed. Ellen will be on your side anyway. She's always wanted a cat."

Despite the family's initial protestations, Tabitha had come to stay. Her days of stealing sausages were over. Now she spent most of her well-fed life on Storm's bed, which the rest of the family often pretended not to notice, and the remainder on her blanket in the laundry when they did.

Each Saturday since then Peter had accompanied Storm to the Village. Several people had called her Ellen, and Peter had told them it was a misprint. Could they please call her Storm instead? Young men were always coming around as well, but reading the clear warning in Peter's eye, quickly realised their attempt to pick up the hot artist chick would go seriously awry while her blasted brother was around.

When Storm discovered there were other followers of the Way meeting in the local school hall every Sunday, she had asked to go along. Peter, who didn't trust Christian young men any more than he trusted the potential suitors lining up at the Village, went along with her, first with the greatest reluctance, and more recently with a willingness which surprised the rest of the family no end. Now he had begun to attend church every Sunday with an increasing eagerness, much to Storm's delight.

To Ellen it was the last straw. Peter was slowly being sucked into a black hole, and she was powerless to prevent it. She read the feelings behind his eyes every time he gazed at Storm, but saw none of that adoration returned by the girl herself. *He's going to be hurt so badly,* she thought. *She's using him. Now she's got him going all religious. I hate it, and I hate her!* All that week Ellen had allowed her anger to grow in silence, until by the following Sunday it had reached truly alarming proportions.

STORM DANCING

That Sunday morning Ellen was absent from breakfast, and Basa went to her bedroom, supposing she must not be feeling well. The girl was sitting up on the end of her bed, and although she wasn't crying, there were tear streaks down her cheeks and an expression on her face to match. Basa sat beside the bundle of misery and put her arm around her shoulder.

She was about to ask what was wrong when Ellen exploded at full volume. "I'm going to live somewhere else!"

"Where would that be, darling?"

"Anywhere."

Basa said nothing, and started to rub her back. More would come soon enough, and it did.

"I used to be a part of this family," Ellen cried, "now I'm just the baby sister no one wants. It's Storm this, Storm that, and now Peter's her willing slave. You're all her willing slaves."

Tears were streaming down her face now, but her eyes were burning with fury. "She was my baby sister, now she's telling me what to do. And all this religion. Now she's sucking Peter into it. Can't you see? She's taken over his brain. She's taken over the whole family. And she's so bloody smart. I taught her to... to go to the toilet, and now she's trying to teach me stuff. She hates me."

Basa waited until reason and logic had a chance, which meant listening to a lot more words which carried the same clear message. Eventually the time came, and Ellen sat silent and tearful watching her mother.

"Ellen, you're my flesh and blood," Basa said quietly. "I could never love you one bit less. Love isn't like a pie at the table, Ellen, the more guests the less each serve. It was because of you that Storm came to stay with us. If you hadn't taught her to go to the toilet, I would have stabbed her with an injection, and uncle Brian would have come and taken her away in the police car. Would you really have wanted that to happen?"

Ellen was silent at first, then she shook her head.

"You've been a wonderful sister to Storm," Basa continued, "and she loves you very much. I know you know that. She's always been older, Ellen. Now her mind is catching up with her age, and this has made it very hard for you. Her faith is something we all find a bit strange, but it hasn't made her a harder person to love, just the reverse in fact."

"Why does she have to be so ... so... damn clever?" Ellen balled her fists.

"You're clever too, Ellen, but you're younger. Storm has already lived another life before she came here, and although she can't remember it, some of the skills she learnt when she was your age are still there."

"There's nothing left from what she was," Ellen said indignantly.

"Yes there is, think about it," Basa said gently. "What can Storm do that we've never taught her?"

There was a long pause. Finally Ellen was struck with a new thought. "She can draw," she said in a surprised voice. "We never taught her to draw."

"That's right. Someone else taught her. She had all that learning before she came here."

"Peter's head over heels crazy about her. He doesn't care about me anymore." Ellen said with a sob.

"I think you might have misread the way Peter is with Storm," Basa comforted, attempting to soften the jealousy in her offspring. "You're completely wrong about him not caring for you. There's something you may be missing, Ellen. Of course Peter loves her, we all love her, but he sees himself as her protector, and he is. He would be your protector too if you were in the slightest danger." She stroked Ellen's hair gently.

"For all Storm's cleverness she's incredibly naïve," Basa continued. "She's just as likely to trust a stranger and get into his car, even though we've told her heaps and heaps of times that's not what you do. She takes people at their face value. It's been getting a bit better lately, but she's still so vulnerable and Peter knows it. That's why he goes with her, to keep nasty people away."

"She's taken over his brain." Ellen stamped her foot.

"Taken over Peter's brain?" Basa smiled. "You're not serious. The boy who comes eleventh in the state? No, Peter is very much the master of his own brain. So are you, my clever Ellen. By the time you have had as much teaching as Storm, you will be every bit her equal. You remember the parent interviews this year? Your teacher told me you have the vocabulary of an eighteen year old, and a reading age of eleven. If you spent more time in books and less time in the television, your reading age would increase dramatically."

"Yeah, I know, Mum, but you're wrong about Peter," Ellen said with complete assurance. "I've watched the way he looks at her. It just goes over her head. She doesn't realise what she's doing to him. You can't blame him, she's got a really hot body."

"Basa laughed. "She's pretty, but she's not the only pretty girl in this family. Come here and cuddle me."

Ellen came and cuddled. She felt better now she had poured it all out. She had never thought that some of Storm's cleverness had come from things she learnt before she arrived. But her mother was wrong. Peter was in love with Storm. It takes a girl to know, she thought to herself, forgetting her mother was another member of the same species and gender.

Basa went back to the kitchen and made herself a cup of tea. She knew very well how her son felt about Storm. Everyone could see it except the girl herself apparently, and Ellen was particularly perceptive. She could well understand her jealousy, because initially she had suffered from the same complaint herself. How on earth would this end? The last thing she wanted was any member of her family to get hurt, including

Storm. Even if the girl felt the same way, how could they ever get married? She gave a soft groan and went to find Andrew.

❊ ❊ ❊

Christmas came joyfully and its glow lingered until New Year. The family watched the fireworks on television rather than joining the enormous crowds squeezed into every metre of harbour foreshore, and enjoyed them very much.

Midway through January, Peter learned from the newspaper - and the same day by letter, that he had been accepted into the faculty of Medicine at Sydney University. The family were overjoyed, and it was Andrew's idea to have a party. Peter said it would be wonderful, but his heart sank. He didn't like parties overmuch. The thought of having one in his own home didn't thrill him at all, but he knew his parents wanted to celebrate his achievement and he wasn't going to stop them.

"A great idea," Ellen said. There are some really cool guys in your year."

"Name one." Peter sounded cross.

"Harry the hunk," Ellen said, bright-eyed. "I've heard the girls on the bus talking about him. I go to high school this year and—"

Peter turned a very serious face towards his sister. Gerard Harris was 'Harry the hunk' to girls who didn't know him and 'Gerry the jerk' to anyone who did. "He's a complete loser," he interrupted. "One thing sure, he's not invited. I doubt he even passed. His father's a barrister, but the jerk thinks more about the bedroom than the bar."

"We get the picture," Andrew said quickly. "We don't want any more description of Mr. Harris' activities."

"I do," Ellen said enthusiastically.

"No you don't." Three voices spoke in unison.

Storm Dancing

Although Storm helped in the preparations every bit as much as the other members of her family, they all noticed her enthusiasm for the evening was even more sadly lacking than Peter's. In the end she told everyone she would stay in her room, because the thought of meeting all those new people made her feel tired and uncomfortable. Peter said that was a great idea, because he didn't want Storm meeting any of his male classmates. Some of them would take instant advantage of her naiveté, the others would distract her from her studies. Something deep within his soul rebelled at the thought of Storm with a boyfriend.

The night of the party arrived, and an hour later the whole house was filled with guests. Ellen was chatting with the guys who were willing to spend time talking to a primary schooler, and the girls were chatting with the other ones who weren't. Peter moved from guest to guest making polite conversation and thanking them for their congratulations, which were sometimes more politically correct than sincere.

There was a knock at the door. Peter opened it to find Gerard Harris standing there with a carton of coolers in his hand, and by the smell of him, another one in his stomach. Harris, needless to say, had not been invited, and if Peter had been able to read his mind on the spot he would have slammed the door in his face. Harris had spent the afternoon watching porn and drinking booze with a few of his selected sleazy mates. The porn had increased his lust, and the booze had decreased his restraint. By the time the last movie had finished and the last can had been drunk, he was desperate to find some willing girl on whom to unleash the depravity he had nurtured all afternoon. He had decided to go to Craig's party purely on impulse, which was the way he decided anything. Craig was rumoured to have a really hot sister who presented hitherto untried opportunities, and he knew Craig would hate it if he scored. He liked the idea from both angles. Besides, it was the only party going, and Harris hated even the thought of returning home. Might run into his old man, an encounter to be avoided at all costs.

"What are you doing here, Harris?" There was not a trace of friendliness in Peter's voice.

"You forgot to invite me, no hard feelings. Out of the way, Craig. There's girls I want to meet."

"Not with the coolers," Peter countered. "There's no alcohol at this party, except the stuff you've already drunk before you came here."

"It's a free country, Craig. People can drink if they want to," Harris sneered, refusing to put down his burden.

"It stays where it is on the path or you don't come in. Didn't you hear my son?" Andrew, who was now standing behind Peter, wore an expression that gave Harris cause for pause.

"Only trying to liven up the party. No problem, I'll just pick it up when I leave," Harris said in a belligerent tone.

He pushed past Andrew and Peter heading for the nearest group of girls, who took one look at the newcomer and melted away into the crowd. They subtly reconfigured themselves around those who would not hesitate to tell Gerry the jerk where to go. In fact wherever he went, a small but definite space opened up around him. He made his way over to the drinks, grabbed a diet coke from Basa's hand without so much as a 'thank you' and turned his back on her to drink it. Jerk, thought Peter who was watching him out of the corner of his eye. Throwing the empty can into the ice bucket with all the other unopened ones, Harris turned around in search of his next female victim.

He was just about to make a move towards Robyn Fields in transit from the nibbles table, when he spied Storm in the hallway. The girl was returning from the bathroom before going to bed, so she was wearing her dressing gown. She noticed Harris staring at her and smiled at him. Harris smiled back. The girl was even hotter than he had been led to believe. Storm opened the door to her bedroom and went inside. Harris needed no further invitation. Girls wearing dressing gowns were ready to get into bed naked, and the smile told him she was just gagging for it. Hot sex was mere seconds away. Harris detached himself from the space around him, and moved down the hall towards the door Storm had disappeared into. Without waiting for an invitation, he strode inside just as the girl was in the act of untying her dressing gown before getting into bed. Gerry could feel his body preparing for the sex to come.

He shut the door behind him and launched. "It's gonna be brilliant, babe."

Storm turned round to see a stranger striding towards her. The next second his arms were inside her gown around her naked body, and his face close to her own. She was petrified, unable to move or cry out. Interpreting her lack of resistance as proof positive that he had correctly interpreted her mood, Harris wrenched her head towards him, covered her mouth with his own, and shoved his tongue down her throat. At first Storm thought she was going to pass out with fright. She could feel her heart hammering in her chest, felt the foul thing in her mouth. She clamped her teeth down hard on it. Harris tried to pull his tongue out and found he couldn't. Storm bit harder, feeling his grip slacken as she did. Harris brought his knee up viciously into her stomach. Storm fell over backwards onto the floor, holding her stomach and crying in pain.

Harris spat blood out of his mouth and came slowly towards her, his face black with hate. "Bish!... gunna urt oo!"

He raised his boot to deliver what would have been a serious injury, but the blow never fell. Peter's left fist landed like a cannon ball in his stomach, and when he bent over in agony, Peter's right fist delivered a sizzling blow to his jaw. Harris sailed over Storm's body and landed amidst the wreckage of the bedside cabinet. Storm struggled up from the floor and hid behind Peter, pressing hard against his back, her arms gripping him so tight around the chest he could hardly breathe, let alone deal with Harris, who was beginning to get up from the wreckage. Things might have gone ill, but right at that second Basa strode into the room. She sized up the situation instantly, walked over to Harris who had just got to his feet, and delivered a withering slap to his left cheek which knocked him straight back into the wreckage again. You could have heard the sound of that blow across the street. Harris struggled to his feet even more groggy than before.

"That's for attempting to rape my daughter," Basa said in a very level 'quiet-before-the-nuclear-explosion' sort of voice.

Harris stared at her in a state of utter bewilderment. No girl had ever bitten his tongue, and no woman had ever slapped his face. His first thought was to hit back, but the rage in Basa's eyes put paid to that idea. He could see her left arm preparing to deliver another dose of the same medicine. The room was going round in a most disconcerting fashion. Somehow the situation had spiralled out of control.

"She wanned secs... ricked me.. I'm gunna sue," he spluttered hatefully.

"Andrew get the police," Basa called over her shoulder to Andrew who had just come into the room.

There were a large number of other faces in the doorway behind him.

She turned to the groggy young man. "Open your mouth so I can see what damage has been done. Personally I hope she's bitten it in half. Come on, I'm a doctor. Stop behaving like a baby."

Harris half opened his mouth. Basa grabbed hold of his lower and upper jaw and yanked it wide. He gave a yell of pain.

"You need some attention," Basa snapped. "Your tongue requires a stitch."

"A sicccs? No!" Harris said, horrified.

"Pathetic," Basa growled. "Come on."

Grabbing Harris by the arm, she propelled him out of the room and slammed the door shut behind her. Storm began to sob her heart out, and Peter could feel her warm tears running over his neck and down his back. Hatred and rage the like of which he could never have imagined drove those blows to Harris. He had wanted to smash his face to pulp, laugh to the music of his screams, kick him to death as he lay there stunned on the floor. Only Storm's arms like steel across his chest had prevented him.

Minutes before, he had glanced up to see Harris disappearing into Storm's bedroom and torn down the corridor like a maniac. He had flung open the door to find her lying on the floor half naked and crying in pain. If he had been carrying a knife, Harris would be wearing it through the heart, he knew. Once he had thought himself totally above such actions, now he realised to his horror that he was not.

He heard Storm's soft voice in his ear. "Peter, you stopped him... I would have been..."

More broken-hearted sobbing followed. Peter covered her hands and arms with his own and held them against him. "Don't think about it," he said. "Just don't think about it. I saw you lying on the floor and I went crazy. I wanted to kill him, Storm. I can't bear anyone hurting you. You stopped me. I wanted to kill him."

"I love you, Peter... I love you Peter." For a long time that was all she could say. He felt her arms relax a little. "Peter, can you turn round, please?"

Peter turned round. Her dressing gown was only on her arms and draped over her back. She pressed her naked body hard against him, her face into his neck.

"Hold me, Peter. I want to feel your clothes against me. I want to remember your clothes against me, not his. I want to feel your arms around me, on my skin. I don't want to remember his. Can you put your arms on my skin? Do you understand?"

"Yeah, I guess."

He slipped his arms inside her dressing gown and pressed her tight against him, doing his best not to peek at what he was holding. Her skin was soft and warm. He prayed that neither Ellen nor his parents would choose this instant to come into the room.

After a while Storm relaxed her grip around his back. "Close your eyes and let go, Peter. Thank you. Open now."

Storm had wrapped her dressing gown around her and was tying the cord. "Can you sit with me a while? I don't want to see anyone else."

He helped her over to her bed and sat close to her, his arm around her waist.

For a long time she sat there, sad and silent. "Are all the men out there like him, Peter? Is that what they all want to do to me?"

"No, Storm. Not everyone's a swine like Harris."

"I feel so dirty. His eyes were burning with hate, Peter. He would have killed me, he wanted to."

She shuddered. Peter tightened his grip around her waist, drawing her close against him.

"I read about people like him in the Children's Bible, but it wasn't real then. It's real now." She turned a pair of large, sad eyes towards him. "Peter, part of me is like that too. I knew I was hurting him, but I didn't want to stop... I'm ashamed of myself. Jesus was ashamed of me."

There was another long pause. Storm's words had shocked him, because he recognised the truth in them. He remembered how he had felt, and how it had frightened him. "But Jesus can forgive you, can't he?" he said at length.

"Of course, Peter. He has already." She shuddered again, reached out and gripped the hand around her waist with both of hers, pulling his arm even tighter around her. "You held me. I must remember. You've got a pen in your pocket and it stuck into me. I'm glad you had a pen in your pocket, Peter."

Their conversation was interrupted by Ellen who burst through the door and launched herself at Peter. "You're awesome!" She exclaimed, scrambling up on to the bed next to him and giving him a ferocious squeeze. "You really fixed him. Mum had him in the surgery for ages. There was this scream – did you hear it? I thought Mum had torn out his tongue with forceps, or castrated him with a scalpel. Dad was on the phone, so I rushed into the surgery to see what she was doing."

"Ellen that really isn't helping," Peter said gently. "We're both feeling a bit feral towards Harris right now. What did happen?"

"Mum put some iodine and alcohol mixture on his tongue. He's such a baby, bullies often are, aren't they? Then Dad came in and Harris said a whole lot of stuff about telling the police that Storm was a slut, and that she had begged him for you-know-what, and he was in her bedroom by invitation when he was viciously attacked by the family. He said it was a conspiracy against him because we all hated him, and he'd make sure our name was – then he used some words that Mum doesn't let me say."

"Mum stood for all that?" Peter asked.

"Dad butted in and told him he'd rung his father, not the police. Harris went a funny colour and said he wasn't waiting round for that old bore. He tried to get off the table, but Mum stuck a needle in his arm and he went down like a dead pig. She said it was a sedative because she needed to stitch his tongue, but she was really angry. I could tell by the way she stabbed him with the needle and wrenched it out."

"What's happened to the party?" Peter said. "It's all quiet out there."

"Most of the girls shot through with their phones in their hand tweeting like mad to their friends," Ellen explained. "Some of Peter's mates stayed around because they said they wanted to give Harris some post-operative treatment on the front lawn to help him remember the party, but dad shooed them off."

"Where are Mum and Dad now?" Peter asked.

"With Barrister Harris. He looks dreadful, and he keeps saying "I'm so sorry, I'm so sorry" like he's got a software glitch. Oh, and Mum asks if you two would like to come out so he can glitch all over you as well."

Storm shook her head. "I'll go," Peter said. "Can you stay with Storm?"

Ellen nodded. When Peter had left she moved closer, and after a little hesitation put both arms around her.

"I've been jealous," she said, "about you and Peter. I'm sorry. I'm really glad he got here in time before—"

Storm gently covered Ellen's lips with her hand. "Before anything happened. Yes, he's a wonderful brother – and you're my wonderful sister." She stroked Ellen's hair gently. "I've missed you. Peter saved me this evening, but don't you remember, you're the one who saved my life? Do you think for a single second that I don't love you too? You gave me my name, Ellen. Think about it. Only a grown up can name their child, but you named me. That makes something very special between us." She wrapped the girl into her arms and kissed her softly on top of her head. Ellen began to cry quietly. Storm felt her head nod up and down and her arms tighten.

Finally she stopped and looked up into Storm's face. "Harris is such a bastard. I would have—"

"That doesn't help, Ellen."

"Help for what?"

"For me to forgive him."

"Forgive him?" Ellen said incredulously. "Who wants to forgive him? I'll make sure every girl I know finds out what you did. He'll be tongueless before the end of the year and serve him right."

"Ellen," Storm said softly, stroking the girl's hair, "just imagine if I kept this hatred that's been planted in my heart tonight and grew it, grew it, day after day. Who do you think would get hurt? Harris? Not at all. It would be me, Ellen. Forgiveness is the only thing that cancels hatred out, like Jesus did for me."

Ellen rolled her eyes, but only a little bit. The usual stinging comment about Storm's obsession with following the Way was missing too.

"I'll think about that," she said softly.

STORM DANCING

Outside in the lounge room Barrister Rowland Harris was still in the act of apologising. "There have been others," he said sadly, with the air of a man who found the words very difficult to say. "I fear the girls involved were afraid to say anything. No doubt my son blackmailed or threatened them. I will have to get to the bottom of those incidents now." He sighed, "he's been pampered and indulged all his life. Dorothy would deny him nothing, and this is the way he rewards us. A long dose of juvenile correction would do him good. I take it the young lady would not be up to hearing my apology?"

Peter shook his head. "Storm's – Helen's too upset right now. I'll convey the message tomorrow when she's feeling less shaken up."

He's starting to come round, Mr. Harris." Basa returned to the room after a short visit to the surgery. "I'll bring him in here."

"Then I'll take him home," Harris said grimly, "and I hope his ears aren't anesthetised because I'm going to fill them with some words he won't like. Now before I go, I say again, if there is anything at all I can help you with in the future, I want you to call me. It would ease the burden on my conscience. That sounds selfish, but I'm in your debt and I know it. You could have taken other action tonight and escalated this incident to the detriment of my whole family. I find it hard to express gratitude. Please don't forget."

Harris was still groggy when he staggered into the room with Basa's fist clamped round his arm. His father gave him a withering glare, and propelled him down the hall, out the door and into the large Mercedes parked in the gutter outside. Certain loud and appropriate descriptions of his behaviour floated through the evening air before the car doors were shut.

With Harris and his father gone, Basa went into Storm's room for a mother-daughter talk and shooed Ellen out. A full half hour went by before she came out again, followed by the girl herself. Andrew came over to her and gave her shoulder a rub. Perhaps she wouldn't want a man hugging her just yet. Storm read the expression in his face and threw her arms around him.

"Thank you, Daddy." The words were muffled in his chest. "Peter protected me. He was so strong. If he hadn't been there ... " Once again the tears flowed, shorter now. Soon Storm was able to sit down at the breakfast room table with the rest of the family and eat some of the large quantity of left over party food. Ellen was quiet, which was unexpected, and Peter was quiet, which was. It took quite a while to clean up the remains of the party and get the house back to its usual state, and everyone was tired by the time they did.

Peter went to bed and fell into a deep sleep almost instantly. The sun was well in the sky when he began to wake up, turned over, and to his astonishment found he was not alone. Curled up on top of the covers beside him, her head on a cushion from the chair, wearing her dressing gown and sound asleep was Storm. Peter had never come to consciousness faster. He lay there watching her, deeply aware of how beautiful she was, his heart beating madly. He saw her eyes open and stay staring at him, neither laughing nor serious, as though she was drinking in the sight of his head on the pillow, content beyond all measure to be where she was. For what seemed a long, long time she lay there, simply watching him, saying not a word. At last she reached out and stroked his hair tenderly.

"Woke up," she said softly. "Bad dream. Felt frightened. Needed you near me. Not frightened when I'm near you." She uncurled and slid off the bed. "I'll go now before Ellen wakes up. She has such a silly imagination. You're a wonderful brother. I love you, Peter."

She stumbled awkwardly out of the room and closed the door softly behind her. Peter lay there staring at that door for an awfully long time. Ellen's imagination was nowhere as silly as Storm supposed.

CHAPTER 20

James Hunt left his half empty schooner on the bar and walked out into the cool Redfern night. King street was ablaze with light from the pavement signs advertising a plethora of culinary delights, right down to where the road bent away to the left. Traffic was heavy. It was always heavy down King Street, no matter what time of day or night. On the opposite side of the road a busker was bruising the ears of every passing pedestrian with a murdered version of 'What a Woman What a Night' delivered at competitive volume to the nightclub further down the street playing disco music. A gaggle of girls passed him going in the opposite direction, wearing tight blue tops and tiny short jeans with ragged edges. Their long, bare skinny legs sported black high heeled boots on their long, skinny feet.

It had been another fruitless search. The theatre had been just two blocks away, but no one could even remember it. Now, as part of the gentrification of Sydney's inner suburbs, it had been turned into a series of yuppie apartments, rendered all the more ridiculous because the old theatre façade still remained. Not only was it filthy with paint peeling off the cheap red brickwork, it was still covered with the remains of posters advertising the delightful shows which its former patrons enjoyed within. Small sections of discoloured buttocks and faded costumes still darkened the faded paper strips which had resisted the efforts of determined hands to rid the wall of their anachronistic presence.

MAC CUSITER

Perhaps he had mistaken the place, there was every chance he had considering the bender he and his mates had been on that night. One more visit and he would put the task into the too hard basket and leave it there. Pity, the scent of a story lingered despite the lack of evidence. It was night when he had gone to see the play, a complete waste of time. Some indecipherable gibberish, its genesis in the playwright's scotch rather than his senses, but she had been on stage, the naked woman who bore the amazing likeness to the teenage artist. By all accounts he was chasing a doppelganger in any case. He had turned the corner by now, the converted theatre in front of him on the opposite side of the road, its brightly lit entrance contrasting with its darkened paper strewn façade. This had to be the place. He crossed over towards it. The lights from a passing car swept the dismal scene, illuminating the drab wall in all its faded glory. In that harsh, moving light the loose ends of shredded paper strips seemed to wave at him as their shadows moved along the filthy brickwork. He reached up idly and tore another piece away, a civic act which should have been completed prior to a damn good coat of paint. Either that or demolish the whole ridiculous thing and start again with an entrance which matched the modern apartments behind it.

He glanced disinterestedly at the small fragment in his hand. No trace of a picture discoloured its surface, only part of one word - DEMAR and the remains of another letter which could have been a P or another R. He screwed the piece up and threw it into a rubbish bin which some thoughtful council had left on the side of the road at just the right place. Demar, he thought, and purely at a whim, pulled out his phone, selected the internet, and typed the word in. A list of possible matches scrolled down the screen, all nonsense, but the sixth one down caught his attention. Demarra, Rachel, actress, pictures, filmography. He clicked on the site. After a few minutes a picture of Ms. Rachel Demarra popped up on the screen.

The two young men who were about to enter their apartment turned in astonishment to see a stranger dancing and shouting for joy on the street not far from them, waving his mobile phone over his head like a ribbon on Australia day.

Hunt returned to his car in a state of great excitement. Someone had scoured a long, deep scratch along its length with a broken bottle.

Obviously the gentrification process in this part of town was not complete. Even this didn't dampen his spirits. What a long shot, but it had paid off. Arriving at his home in Cherrybrook in far less time than would be indicated by the speed suggestions on the side of the road, Hunt fired up his computer and typed in the name. There she was, Rachel Demarra, Australian actress now resident in LA, list of films and their reviews, once voted ninth most beautiful woman in the world – yeah, she was quite a stunner. Her bio followed. Born in Kirribilli to John and Helen Demarra, only child, studied at NIDA, reputation for appearing nude in plays by H. Donahue, one daughter Felicity who died tragically one month after being electrocuted during a holiday in Queensland, never regained consciousness. Mother left for the States after that, settled in LA where her career as an actress began to take off. No pictures of Felicity. Damn, doppelganger, yet the likeness was uncanny. He stared at the pictures of Rachel, either taken years ago or touched up. No woman held her age that well, but you never knew in these days of modern medicine. Ah, back to the drawing board. It had been a good hunch.

His finger moved the pointer over to the little red cross on the top right hand corner of the browser. He was about to close the application when his phone beeped. A date and time had flashed up on its small screen, his first appointment tomorrow morning.

Date and time! He was losing focus, the devil was always in the details. He scrolled back through the biopic, studying more closely the information he had previously disregarded. Now that was unusual. Rachel Demarra had left Australia the very day her daughter had been cremated at Northern Suburbs Crematorium Sydney, the day after she had died in Queensland. All done with unnecessary haste, or was he simply refusing to admit he had been following a dead lead? Hunt closed the website and opened another, one which required a password acquired through his profession. Being a reporter did have some advantages. In a few minutes he was reading a copy of Felicity Demarra's death certificate. Death had occurred at 3:45 a.m., Southport Hospital, certificate signed by one Dr. D. Ferris. The body must have been transported to Sydney almost immediately in order for her to be cremated the very next day. A little more searching and he had the time of the service, 3:00 p.m. It would require some canny organisation to arrange a cremation less than thirty six hours after a death. Perhaps the actress knew someone helpful. Beautiful women often knew someone helpful.

He was chasing shadows.

He closed the web page and opened another. Doctor David Ferris, Senior lecturer in neurophysiology at Sydney University, neurologist at Westmead hospital Sydney. What was he doing in a Gold Coast hospital ward at three a.m. in the morning? Perhaps he was her lover, and may have long since taken on the role of Felicity's doctor. That would explain it, but the speed of the whole process was unusual. Time to interview a certain Doctor David Ferris. He read further. Dr. Ferris had been engaged in research before his untimely death by drowning on the night of a severe storm which struck Sydney. Damn and blast. Another dead end, literally. He searched for and read the account of the drowning, a brief mention amongst the other folk who had perished on that terrible night. Where to go now? After he had written his current article for the Voice he might spend the weekend up in the Gold Coast.

✳ ✳ ✳

The next day Harry Sloane ambled into the cubicle just as Hunt was finishing his article. "Peaceful around here with George down in Melbourne, isn't it?" he laughed. "How's it going?" Some article about possums. George likes animals. You'll probably get a promotion."

Hunt grimaced. "I doubt it. You know the bloke who was advertising possum relocation services?"

"You thought it was a bit odd as I recall," Sloane said, "especially at ten dollars a service. His competitors were charging a hundred."

"Turns out he would pick the possums up in a cage, take them home and wring their necks," Hunt said wearily. "To make matters worse, he threw all the bodies into his neighbour's back yard. Delightful specimen of humanity with a pathological hatred of possums as well as a grudge against his neighbour."

Sloane whistled. "Serious stuff. Managed to get some good evidence?"

Hunt laughed. "All captured on infra-red camera. What's more, the bloke turns out to be none other than Shire Councillor McLean."

"Better bury the article," Sloane said alarmed. "That guy is mates with our beloved editor. I don't want to find you shoved in some backyard with your throat cut."

Hunt grunted. "Too late, mate. I've just sent it to layout. Made the front page at last."

George arrived back the next day to read the headline on page one:

GET YOUR POSSUMS WHACKED FOR $10
TERMINATOR ON COUNCIL PAYROLL

He hit the roof. "Gutter journalism," he bellowed, loud enough to frighten everyone in the building. Thundering obscenities down the corridor, he burst into Hunt's cubicle and lunged at the man. Hunt, warned by the racket, was waiting. Curling his boot inside the metal rubbish bin, he sent it flying into George's face. George jumped backwards, blood pouring from his nose, and hit his head on the wall. Hunt picked up his office chair and swung it hard into George's stomach as he staggered towards him. George collapsed on the floor, groaning.

Hunt planted his boot on George's wrist. "Now George," he said, "I take it my employment has been terminated. I've got some more gutter journalism for you. Remember those nature walks you like to take in Pennant Hills Park? I thought I'd follow you one day, just to see your taste in roses."

"Bastard," George spluttered, but made no attempt to get up. His wrist was becoming very painful.

"I've got some lovely pictures," Hunt went on. "If you ever do anything I don't like, you'll find yourself on the front page of a decent newspaper. I'm sure a certain Mayor would be really interested to discover that his wife shares the same taste in roses as you do."

George turned as pale as possible for a man in his reduced circumstances. Hunt removed his boot from George's wrist, picked up his briefcase and left the building to the sound of anonymous applause coming from nearly every other cubicle.

Chapter 21

Being without a job at just that time was an advantage. Hunt booked a flight for the Gold Coast the next day and treated himself to a well-deserved lunch.

Arriving home, he switched on his computer and began searching for the hotel in which Felicity Demarra died. No doubt it would be recorded in police files, but he couldn't access those. He tried local papers, not a mention, Brisbane dailies, not a mention, community notice boards, not a mention. He was about to throw in the towel, when just before midnight he struck oil. A local Gold Coast trade journal made a passing reference to a young girl being electrocuted at the poolside. No name was given, but it had named the hotel and the date. The article went on to plead for more stringent safety standards around swimming pools in Gold Coast hotels. It was a long shot, but now he had a possible location.

He caught the morning flight to the Gold Coast, and arrived at Southport hospital around midday. Could he please speak to the resident neurologist? That would be Doctor Travers, and no, he couldn't. Doctor Travers was currently operating. Perhaps Mr. James would care to come back tomorrow? Mr. James had no intention of coming back tomorrow, so he said he would wait. Wandering around the wards he discovered that Travers always did his rounds in the early afternoon after his regular operation schedule. Hunt went down to the canteen and bought himself a pie and a cup of coffee. He threw the coffee away after one mouthful, and went over to the machine for a soft drink. An hour later he returned to the nurse's station on the neurological ward. None of the staff currently employed could remember a young girl who had been electrocuted, so Hunt waited for Travers who arrived an hour later.

Travers was a taciturn man at the best of times, and when he discovered who Hunt was and what he wanted, he became positively hostile and uncommunicative. Did he remember the young woman? Grunt. Did he remember treating her? Grunt. Did he remember the night she died? The question obviously stirred an unpleasant memory, because Travers turned to Hunt as though he was contemplating how much he would enjoy removing his brain.

"I wasn't on duty that night," he growled. "Some other doctor from Sydney was. When I turned up in the morning the girl had died and been taken off the ward. I'm not responsible for what happened."

"Doctor Ferris was scheduled on the ward that evening?" Hunt asked politely, ignoring the thinly veiled animosity.

"Who's Doctor Ferris?" Travers growled again. "I lodged a serious complaint with management, but as you would expect from this apology for an administration I have not had the courtesy of a reply."

"Had you ever heard of Doctor Ferris prior to that night?"

"This nonsense is over."

Travers picked up a clipboard from a peg in the nurse's station and strode into the ward. Clearly that line of investigation had reached an end, but it hadn't been entirely unfruitful.

His next visit was to the hotel where Felicity could have died. Following on from his experience at the hospital he anticipated the same unfriendliness raised to a higher power. Exactly the opposite occurred. In response to his initial question, the concierge requested the manager to come down to the front desk. Within minutes he was introduced to Mr. Kevin Nolands who couldn't have been more affable if he tried.

"I've never heard of the event you speak of, Mr. Hunt," Nolands said apologetically, "but that's hardly surprising, seeing as I was employed here about six months after that date. No, I don't believe any of our duty managers were here either, although you are most welcome to enquire. I can bring all those on duty to the conference room if you wish, and we could convene a meeting in half an hour. The rest you could meet tomorrow." He smiled effusively. "You've come a long way, and probably did not expect to have to stay over. Please allow me to offer the hospitality of our resort at no cost to yourself. We're very conscious of maintaining an impeccable reputation, Mr. Hunt, and will do whatever we can to assist you. From what you describe it was a terrible business."

Hunt met with around twenty staff exactly half an hour later. Not one of them was employed at the hotel when the incident occurred. Hunt declined the meeting tomorrow, thanked the manager for his courtesy, and returned to his room. This had to be the place alright. After freshening up he decided to visit the fateful pool where Felicity had met her lingering death. Peering out from his window he could see it directly below him with its tree lined perimeter. He caught the lift down and walked out on the paving which covered the poolside. A few adults were stroking up and down its length, obviously keeping up their fitness, and some children were swimming in the shallows. A couple of lovers were playing in the deeper end, diving together and coming up the same way. Hunt walked the length of the pool and turned towards the trees which lined the area. On the other side, tending the garden, was an older man in overalls, a pruning hook stuck in his belt. He was raking leaves in an attempt to prevent them blowing into the pool. It was a long shot, but then, one long shot had already paid off.

"Hi," he said, "My name's James. I'm a reporter from Sydney, making some enquires about a girl who was electrocuted not far from this spot some years ago. I take it you can't remember the incident? No one else can."

"James, is it?" The gardener paused in his raking and stood staring at Hunt with interested eyes. "Well, Mr. James, I usually knock off around six thirty and have a schooner at the bar down the road, perhaps even dinner. It's not as Cordon Bleu as the restaurant here, but then the atmosphere has much to commend it. Perhaps I will see you there."

He went back to raking leaves. Hunt moved away as fast as possible. Once again his long shot had paid off, or at least showed promise. The afternoon dragged slowly, painfully slowly. At six o'clock he had a shower and a shave, dressed casually in the spare set of clothes he had brought just in case, and ambled out of the hotel. The bar down the road turned out to be quite a long way down the road, and by the time he arrived, Hunt could feel the perspiration running down his back. Typical Queensland weather, hot and incredibly humid. He went in and ordered a schooner of light. The bar was crowded, but there were still some tables in the back. The menu boasted steak and your choice of mashed potatoes or chips for fifteen dollars, very reasonable. He ordered another schooner of light, and was raising it to his lips when the gardener came through the door.

He strolled up to Hunt as though he had never seen him in his life, sat down on the nearest barstool, and without turning in his direction gave Hunt his order. "Schooner of Kilkenny dark, steak with mash and I'll see you on that table right at the back."

He vacated the barstool and headed off in that direction. Hunt bought a schooner of some dark liquid with a creamy white head, ordered the steaks, picked up the tag and the beers and headed towards the back to join the man.

"Here," he said, handing the man the beer. "I take it you know something about the incident. How come everyone else seems to have a case of convenient amnesia? Nobody gives a rats arse about some chick who was stupid enough to get herself electrocuted, but not to remember it at all seems a bit strange to me."

The old man took a long drink of the dark liquid, wiped the foam from his upper lip and smiled at him. "Pat Murray at your service, Mr. James. Yes, it does seem a trifle odd, doesn't it? How much do you know?"

Hunt told him.

"You're not doing too good for a reporter, are you?" he chuckled. "Yeah, I was there the morning it happened. Ambulance came, people running around like chooks without heads, panic, panic, panic." He paused and took another long drink. "Not that I could see much, but I know a bit. Mate of Joe Green, police sergeant Joe Green. They called him that morning, see?"

"Anything strike your friend Joe as unusual?"

"He always reckoned someone had interfered with the lights. They used to string 'em up in the trees beside the pool, very pretty. He reckons someone brought 'em down and smashed a few into the bargain."

"Any idea who?" Hunt asked, trying to keep the excitement out of his voice.

"He doesn't, but I have my hunches. Anyway, you want to know why nobody is talking, don't you? Happened at the hearing. The hotel gets told that some woman called Ms. Demartian—"

"Ms. Demarra."

"Always thought it sounded like another planet," Murray nodded, "anyway, her, they gets told she's going to sue the pants off 'em for negligence. Now the hotel chain has their own lawyers, see. They've dealt with this sort of stuff before, and the chain has never had to pay. That's what they think this time, so they don't take all that much notice. But this woman's legal team are feral, high power, and before you know it they've lost the case. Joe had to go to court." He took another drink of the dark liquid. "D' you know the Demartian woman didn't even appear? The hotel lawyers called a few witnesses who said they heard this couple humping in the dark beside the pool that night, and argued it was them who had sabotaged the lights just so they could do it in the dark like. No other evidence, see? So a couple of lovers get carried away near the pool, doesn't excuse the hotel from negligence. Anyway, this is the interesting bit."

He leant forward towards Hunt in a very meaningful way. "The Demartian woman chooses to settle out of court. The hotel chain thinks it's going to be millions, but no, she settles for around a million. Real surprise."

Patrick finished his beer and stared rather longingly into the empty glass. Hunt immediately brought him a fresh one.

"Thank'e," he said, smiling his appreciation. "Everyone thinks it's all over and done with, but now the strange bit happens. Suddenly Head Office starts kicking butt. They sack my mate John Manning and the night manager, Sam somebody, and they start going through the others like a dose of salts, sending them to different resorts all over the map. First we think it's head office being dead scared 'cause they've had the shit kicked out of them by these Sydney barristers and QC's, but no. My mate John has a connection upstairs. He says management have got their knickers in a twist about something else, he doesn't know what, but it's calling the tune and they're running around like little puppets doing as they're told."

He took a long drink, wiped his mouth on his sleeve, and sat back, smiling at the surprised expression on Hunt's face.

"Manning's mate have any idea what scared them?" Hunt asked, his brain working overtime to make sense of what Murray was telling him.

"No. Some mighty powerful show off shore. His mate was scared silly too."

"You said you had a pet theory. Mind if I hear it?"

Their steaks arrived at this point, and for a while Pat was far too busy to reply. Only when the T-bone sat meatless on his plate did he take another pull from his beer, settle back in his chair and speak with a soft, conspiratorial air.

"Joe told me a few things. He said the girl's mother weren't staying with her but with some actor dude from the Hew Hess of Hay. The girl was in a room by herself, see. Mother leaves her daughter to shack up with lover boy. Know what I think? Them lovers in the dark were lover boy and the girl's mum. The hotel reckons they knocked the lights out so they could do it in the dark, but I think different. I think they planned to do her in."

"Murder?" Hunt raised an eyebrow.

"Yeah, murder, and it worked. Got clean away with near on a million dollars."

"But how could they have known the girl would walk into the broken light bulbs?" Hunt asked, trying to think of a plausible explanation himself.

"Search me, mate, but they figured it out somehow," Pat Murray grinned. "Them's two murderers got clean away with it. Joe thinks I'm crazy, but I know different."

Several schooners of dark frothy liquid later, Hunt left a happy and relaxed Pat Murray singing along with the band who had started playing around eight o'clock. The old coot was wrong, surely, because Hunt could see no way of guaranteeing Felicity would walk directly into a death trap, and a hundred reasons why she wouldn't. Who was this other lover? Obviously not Ferris, and that put paid to his previous explanation, unless Demarra was blatantly two-timing him. No doubt those hotel records had been carefully deleted from the database. No point in asking. So far he hadn't learned much, but it was more than enough to keep him interested. His next task was to find out just who Ferris was working with. It was most unlikely that Felicity had met her death by design at the poolside, but not nearly so unlikely that the Demarra woman had employed him to euthanase her. That would explain the haste. Why choose him? Former lover, perhaps. He went back to his room and Googled euthanasia advocates in Australia. Ferris' name wasn't among them.

After an excellent breakfast he checked out without paying a cent. He left a politically correct thank–you note for the Manager, telling him he would recommend the Resort to all his friends, and caught the midday flight back to Sydney. Picking up his car from the long stay car park at Mascot domestic terminal he drove to Westmead hospital.

Westmead hospital was opened in 1978 by the former Premier of New South Wales, Neville Wran. Apart from serving over forty percent of the population of Sydney, it is the largest hospital campus of the University of Sydney Faculty of Medicine. It took Hunt quite a while to locate the medical research centre, and he was surprised at the level of security which had been employed. From the attitude of the woman on the front desk he gathered it was chiefly designed to deter reporters like himself.

"What area of research are you interested in?" she said, eyeing him up and down in an unfriendly manner.

"Neurological."

"We have no current neurological research projects operating, Mr. James. What newspaper did you say you worked for?"

"Freelance. Did a Dr. Ferris ever work here?"

The girl consulted her computer screen grudgingly. "Yes. Why do you want to know?"

"I'm interested in his research team. Who else was he working with?"

"That information can only be released with the approval of the research centre management," she said coldly. "I can give you a form. Excuse me a minute, I have to take this call."

She picked up the phone and turned her back to Hunt, which was fortunate. The computer screen containing the names which he knew he would never obtain, was reflected in the modern black glass panels behind the reception area. It was too small to read at this distance and back to front. Hunt took out his phone and took a picture silently. His phone always took pictures silently.

The woman turned around and put the phone down. "You have a call, Mr. James?"

"Checking my messages. You were saying you had a form?"

"I think it's fair to warn you, management rarely gives information like this to non-academic nosey reporters, Mr. James. In the past we have found their input detrimental to the efficient operation of this research facility."

"If you say so. Ms?"

The girl glared at him. "I need your details for security purposes. You will notice the section where you are required to state the purpose of your visit?" She stabbed the form with her finger. "We have been known to contact the editors of newspapers about the behaviour of their staff."

"Freelance, remember?"

She snatched the form from the counter and waved it in Hunt's face, pointing to a small clear space at the end of the reception desk. Hunt smiled compliance, moved to the space and spent the next ten minutes allowing his imagination free reign. Back in his car he brought up the photo, reversed the image, and enlarged it by spreading his fingers across the screen. It was a little blurry, but perfectly readable.

Project name: Tissue Library 29
Project classification: A RESTRICTED
Project area: Neurological
Project leader: Prof. I. Gilead
Academic
E. Prof. Gerhardt Metzger, d. Head
Dr. D. Ross
Dr. M. Hargraves
Dr. J. Yanac
Dr. D. Ferris
Dr. L. Festerhaus

Diatetics
Dr. R. Lowery
Dr. H. Ammar

Physiotherapy
Dr. P. Krishna
Dr. S. Brown
Dr. P. Cornish

NMR Imaging
Dr. K. Lucknow

More names were obscured by a reflection of the courtyard outside, still he had enough to go on. He decreased the brightness of the image. Now he could make out some more words, enclosed in a box written across the other names in large letters. TERMINATED PREMATURELY. He increased the magnification and adjusted the contrast. No, there was no mistake. The project had been terminated the day after the storm in which Ferris had died. The man obviously played a crucial role, yet he wasn't the leader. Strange, but then the whole thing was strange. A major project involving a large number of highly qualified staff suddenly collapses when one man leaves the team. Ah well, at least he had a few names to check. He started the engine and edged the car out of the parking area. Right now he could use a schooner of pale ale.

CHAPTER 22

Ellen burst through the back door waving her arms around and saying forbidden words at full volume, not an unusual method of attracting her family's attention. She raced across the room to the kitchen sink and threw up in it, instantly raising her performance to Oscar class. Every eye turned. Basa had been at the breakfast table reading, Andrew wiping up in the kitchen. Peter had just arrived from the hall.

"My darling," Basa exclaimed, jumping up, "what on Earth's the matter?"

"Storm's cutting Mr. Macavity apart with a scalpel on the garden table. She's sliced out all his guts and... and... I'm going to be sick again."

Andrew made it to the back door before Peter, and the duo burst out into the backyard. True to description, their neighbour's cat lay on the table, his insides spread all over a newspaper, his organs set aside in neat rows. Storm was measuring the length of his intestines with a ruler. An awful lot of blood and water lay splashed around the area, some of the paper was soaked with it.

Hearing the arrival of her audience, she turned around quite pleased with herself. "Almost two metres," she said proudly. "He was a big boy. Overfed, I'd say."

Andrew placed a handkerchief over his nose. No wonder Ellen had thrown up, the smell nearly turned his stomach. It wasn't exactly carnage, but then it wasn't something the average twelve year old could cope with either. He really hoped Mr. Macavity hadn't walked onto the table by himself at the beginning. All that was needed was Sensitive Sam to poke his head over the fence in search of this pampered pet, and neighbourly relations would hit an all-time low. Storm laid the scalpel down carefully on the newspaper and beamed. Ellen, her eyes averted from the table, appeared with her mother in the distant doorway.

"Ghoul! I want a lock on my bedroom," she shouted.

"Don't be silly, Ellen," Basa said. "What are you doing with Mr. Macavity, Storm?"

It would have been difficult to ask a more superfluous question.

"I found him dead on the road," Storm explained happily. "I wanted to find out what killed him and I did. Look."

Basa, handkerchief in place, came and looked.

"His rib cage was crushed," Storm explained, "and a broken rib pierced his heart. Would have been very quick. There was a lot of haemorrhaging, but I washed it away with the hose. Oh, and his bowel was punctured too, so it smells a bit. Poor Mr. Macavity. Now we can show Mr. Ruston."

"Let me see." Basa came closer to the table, turned over the heart with the scalpel and nodded agreement. "Well done, Storm. Your first autopsy, I'm sure it won't be the last."

"Shall we tell Mr. Ruston now?" Storm asked innocently.

"Ghoul!" Another shout from the backdoor.

"I don't think Mr. Ruston would actually like to see his cat in this condition," Andrew said tactfully. "In fact I think we should clear up the autopsy and give him a decent burial. I'll go and speak to Sam, say we found him in a bit of a mess, and would he like us to bury him in his backyard. He's a bit squeamish, Mr. Ruston, and Amelia is worse. Wrap his remains in a large sheet of clean newspaper, would you Storm? And if you see another dead animal it might be better if you don't perform the autopsy in such a public place. I don't think our Ellen is quite up to an anatomy lesson with real cadavers yet."

From the pallor on Ellen's face when they all came back into the breakfast room, Storm could see Andrew had spoken the truth.

"Sorry, Ellen," Storm said apologetically. "I should have thought a bit more carefully and kept you away."

"Ghoul," Ellen barked. "How many other people have you chopped up for fun? No wonder you can't remember."

Storm turned angrily towards her sister. "Where do you get these stupid ideas?"

"At least I don't go around murdering cats."

"Mr. Macavity was hit by a car," Storm said indignantly. "Do you think I'd have autopsied him if he was still alive?"

"If the shoe fits." Ellen spat caustically.

Storm's name became a metaphor for her face. "You watch too much television," she said angrily. "It's bad for anybody, all those people acting in ridiculous shows. It messes up your mind."

"Not like someone's messed up yours!" Ellen shouted.

For a second Storm stood still, her face black with rage, then all of a sudden it rearranged into a thoughtful smile. Andrew, standing closest, didn't like that smile. Something lay behind it. There was trouble brewing, and he could feel it. Storm had the gentlest personality he had ever encountered, but everyone had limits.

He attempted rescue. "Ellen That was unkind, and you know it. Apologise to Storm."

"No." Ellen stamped her foot.

"Go to your room and come out when you can."

Ellen came out a mere twenty minutes later, mumbled an apology to Storm with fire in her eyes, and descended into a blue funk for the rest of the day.

❋ ❋ ❋

The next day was Sunday. Storm had gone off to the church down the road with Peter as usual. Ellen emerged from her room in a dressing gown around nine thirty, grabbed a muesli bar from the kitchen, and went into the lounge room for her morning dose of MTV before her parents noticed. Andrew and Basa who had just emerged from the hallway after their usual pleasant Sunday sleep-in, caught the torrent of protest coming from the lounge.

"The damn thing's stuffed again!" Ellen shouted.

Sounds of the remote hitting another solid object finished off the tirade. Andrew strode into the room with the face of a man who realises the early bliss of the day has just evaporated like dew in the morning. The TV screen was awash with coloured dots behind which some scantily clad girl was just visible gyrating her body around in a suggestive manner. The confetti might not have improved the picture, but it certainly raised the moral tone.

"I've told you about watching MTV before," Andrew reprimanded. "Change to another channel immediately."

Ellen picked up the remote, reinserted the batteries, scrabbled around a bit until she found the back, and clicked it into place. Every channel was the same.

"The ghoul's stuffed the telly," Ellen fumed loudly.

"Don't be stupid," Andrew groaned. "How could Storm possibly do that? In any case you'll have to watch a DVD instead."

"I hate all my DVD's and you won't let me watch yours," Ellen snapped, sulkily.

"It's a nice sunny day, why don't you go outside?" Andrew said, annoyance still colouring his voice.

"She's probably chopped up Tabitha this time."

"Get over it and grow up," Andrew sighed, going over to the television set.

He spent a good ten minutes fiddling with the aerial connection and anything else which he thought could possibly be wrong, all to no avail. He sighed. Basa came into the room, read the expression on his face, and gave him a hug.

"Why don't we go and have breakfast at the Village café this morning?" she suggested. "We haven't done that for ages."

Andrew kissed her. "Great idea," he said, and they left the room holding hands.

Ellen went back into her room to sulk. After a while she crossed over the hall into Storm's room. Tabitha was curled up in her usual place on the end of the bed.

"Hello Tab," Ellen said, stroking the cat behind the ears. "That's it, go back to sleep. Just forget I was ever here."

An hour later Storm and Peter came home in their usual happy euphoria after being brainwashed, as Ellen called it, by religious rubbish. Storm was singing, as she usually did, and Peter was joining in. A couple of weeks ago he had told the family he had become a follower of the Way. Storm was ecstatic, Ellen furious. Andrew and Basa had shown polite interest.

Ellen was lying on the lounge. She glanced up from the fashion magazine she had found on the kitchen table, and smiled as the two came into the room. "Enjoy your morning?"

"Yes," Storm laughed. "Did you enjoy yours?"

"Oh, yes. More than you know."

There was a tone in Ellen's voice which Storm didn't appreciate, a sort of repressed sassiness, as if to say 'your comeuppance is just around the corner and serve you right.'

Storm went away singing into her bedroom. The singing stopped. Ellen smiled smugly to herself and pretended to concentrate on her magazine.

"What have you done with my books?" Ellen turned her head to find Storm glaring down at her.

"What books?" she asked innocently.

"Don't try that on with me," Storm said, furious. "You've taken them, all the books I read and study with. Where are they?"

"How would I know?" Ellen said sarcastically. "I didn't take them, just like you didn't stuff up the TV."

"You've taken my Children's Bible too," Storm said, barely mastering her temper. "You know how special that book is to me. Give it back."

"Actually it's my Children's Bible," Ellen said. "I threw it in the rubbish where it belongs. There's no point in searching for it. It's all buried in food and yuk now."

STORM DANCING

In two swings of her crutches Storm reached the lounge. Throwing them aside, she grabbed Ellen by the arms and hauled her to her feet, ignoring the loud squeal of protest. Holding her with one arm, Storm raised her hand and delivered a resounding slap to her face with the other. Ellen responded by punching Storm in the stomach. Storm fell onto the floor with Ellen on top of her, trying to free her arms from the older girl's grip so she could avenge her burning cheek. Eventually Storm, who was stronger and heavier than Ellen, managed to roll herself into a commanding position on top of her adversary. Ellen shut her eyes in anticipation of more punishment. At that very instant Peter came into the room.

"Storm, what on earth are you doing?" he said. Going over to the girls he took Storm's arm and lifted her off his sister. Ellen scrambled up from the floor, her face furious.

"She hit me," Ellen yelled. "Her psycho past is coming out now. I'd keep away from her if I were you."

"Why?" Peter said, frowning. "Ellen, what did you do?"

"She's taken all my books," Storm said defensively. "She threw my Children's Bible into the rubbish." Tears budded in her eyes. "That book meant so much to me... and ..." She turned suddenly, snatched up her crutches, and left the room.

Ellen sat down on the lounge again, and picked up the fashion magazine as if nothing had happened.

"Did you?" Peter asked severely. "Why, Ellen?"

Ellen threw the magazine across the floor. "She's stopped my fun, so I stopped hers," she said loudly. "I'm not sorry either."

"I think you should give them back," Peter said. "I don't believe you've thrown the Bible into the rubbish. I know you better than that."

231

"You better believe it," Ellen snapped furiously. "And if the television isn't fixed I'm going to throw the rest of them in there too."

She jumped up from the lounge and stomped into the kitchen. Peter went out into the garden for a breath of fresh air. Ellen's behaviour came as no surprise. He knew how annoyed she was about the television, and he knew she was having trouble with his thinly veiled adoration for Storm. What surprised him was Storm's response. She wasn't perfect after all. In a strange way he felt relieved. He had sometimes entertained the fantasy that she was actually an angel doing penance on earth for some heavenly misdemeanour. He sat down on the swing seat and shut his eyes. Something would have to be done, but what? Suddenly the seat moved. Peter opened his eyes to find Storm sitting next to him, a woebegone expression on her face. She wrapped an arm around his waist.

"Sorry," she whispered. "I behaved like a spoilt child. I'm so sad you had to see it."

Peter stroked her hair. "It's okay," he said. "Ellen deserved it. I'm sure she hasn't damaged your Children's Bible. I don't suppose you could fix whatever you did to the television, could you?"

Storm snuggled her head into his shoulder. "I'm not that repentant," she said softly.

Peter tightened his arm around her waist. There didn't seem to be anything else to say. He pushed the swing seat into a gentle rhythm. The storm had been brief, and now the sun was shining brightly on his world. Peter rested his head against hers and shut his eyes.

Andrew and Basa received an edited report of the morning's events from Peter because he thought they ought to know. As a result Basa went and had a serious talk with Ellen, which lasted all of twenty minutes, and Andrew came in for the last ten to add paternal solidarity to the television deal. They would ring a repair man only if Ellen would agree to certain restrictions, and if she didn't the thing could remain broken for all they cared. Ellen would make a proper apology to Storm and return her books, all of them. She would be careful what she said in future, and the way she said it.

A much more sober and sorrowful Ellen performed these very acts at the dinner table that night, then spoiled it somewhat by saying she knew Storm had wrecked the television and it was going to cost her beloved family a fortune to get it fixed. Storm's big innocent eyes convinced everyone present she was guilty as charged, but how she had managed it remained a mystery.

The man from a local TV servicing company came the very next day. He checked everything inside, checked the integrity of the antenna cable, all to no avail. He did it again. An hour later he knocked on the door of the surgery, rather embarrassed.

"It's all fixed, Dr. Craig," he said. "I'm sorry it's taken so long. No, apart from the call-out fee there's no charge. I'd be too ashamed to ask for it."

"What was the matter?" Andrew asked, coming through the surgery door. "I couldn't find anything wrong at all."

"No, me neither." The serviceman shook his head. "I was about to take the set in to the factory for service when something struck me as odd, so I went back outside and had another squiz at the antenna. It was perfect, except it was pointing exactly the opposite way to all the others in the neighbourhood. It was a little loose on the mast, so I turned it round and tightened it up and all was well. You must get some high winds around here."

"Yes, we do get some significant storms sometimes," Andrew agreed, a smile on his face. "Thanks, Mr. ah... Rogers."

Andrew read the name from the invoice. He paid the eighty dollars, and later on that day while he was taking a break for lunch, he went into the house and found Storm doing maths problems on the desk in her room.

He placed the invoice tactfully in front of her. "For you," he said, "and we won't tell the rest of the family. Now, how did you do it?"

Storm fished out an envelope which she had hidden under a maths book, and handed it to him. "It's all in there. I told him I could settle it, but he insisted on seeing you. The aerial's on a little bent pipe attached to the side of the house. If I stood on your step ladder I could twist it round with a crutch."

"You could have fallen off and hurt yourself." He placed his hand gently on the girl's shoulder. "I know some good things have come out of all this brouhaha with Ellen, but can we give it a rest now? I think she's learned her lesson, and she's going to be watching a good deal less TV." He paused in a sudden thought. "Why do you hate it so much, Storm?"

The girl turned her large brown eyes up towards his face and smiled. "Apart from the effect it was having on Ellen? Do you know, I haven't the faintest idea."

She stood up and hugged him, kissing him softly on his cheek. "Love you Daddy."

"Love you too Storm." Andrew left the room with an envelope in his pocket and a smile on his face.

❋ ❋ ❋

The remainder of the year passed uneventfully. Peter became more and more engrossed in his first year medical degree, Ellen read more books and decided she would like to write one. Storm said she would help. The project lasted for several weeks, and by the time the great novelist had finished, the relationship between the two girls was permanently restored. They would spend hours on end arguing about the plot and rolling all over the lounge room floor laughing together. As Ellen's literary talent blossomed, the television came off a very poor second. Some days it never got turned on at all.

Storm spent a long time reading in preparation for her coming Higher School Certificate year at Sydney Institute, and swapped from chemistry to physics because it related better to mathematics. She was able do quite a lot of the experiments at home, after Andrew had bought her some measuring equipment. She would spend long hours at her desk in her room, plugged in to her music and singing along with it. Tabitha would curl up on her lap when it was cold. How she ever managed to study like that was a mystery to Peter who needed absolute quiet. She still managed to go to the Village to draw people on Saturday mornings, but Andrew would drive her, because it was hard to manage the bus on crutches with her easel. Peter would come and help when he could.

Uncle Brian called in regularly to see the family, and, by order of his chief, to check on Storm. At first a duty, it had long since become a delight. He had come to love the girl every bit as much as her family did.

Peter passed his exams with flying colours, and Storm gained a place in her course for next year at the Institute. Thankfully they accepted her name as Hellen Craig, Australian, living with her family at Shepherds Bush Drive, without raising an eyebrow. Only those students from overseas got the full identity treatment.

The family Christmas was even better than the year before, and Ellen celebrated her thirteenth birthday in January.

Chapter 23

Brian Craig walked into Detective Inspector Ray Wright's office wondering what developments had prompted the summons. "You want to see me, boss?" he asked.

"I do," Wright said grimly. "There's been movement in the stations, Craig, odd movement." He stretched back in his chair. "A short time ago I get this report from our mates at Southport police station in the land of the Banana Benders. Some cove has lodged a complaint about a Mr. James, a Sydney reporter, sniffing around the neurological ward at Southport hospital. I thought that was interesting, so I got a description from a Doctor Travers. Perfect match.

"The veritable James Hunt."

"True. The same James Hunt who has recently lost his job on the Northern Voice. I thank Detective Hansen at Southport for the info, and think this is the last of it. Then I get a routine email from the commissioner's office asking for a detailed report on our superfluous citizen. I made the mistake of sending them all your brother's weekly updates. I forgot that our excellent commissioner is also one of those – what do you call them – followers of the Way. No wonder they sparked his interest." He sighed. "The next day I get a verbal from the man himself."

"Robin Naylor? Commissioner Robin Naylor?" Brian's eyes were wide with astonishment.

"The very same. He's taken a sudden and personal interest in our Ms. Storm. He wants a thorough follow-up on the case, quietly, no fuss." Wright sighed heavily. "And he wants it starting now, which is why you're going to spend tomorrow in sunny Queensland."

"Hunt could have been chasing any old story," Brian objected. "What makes you think it's related to Storm?"

"True, just a hunch. I think Hunt is the sort of person that won't let something lie. Besides which I've got the Commissioner on my tail eager for action, and I want to give him some. It might have nothing to do with the girl, in which case you're going to enjoy a nice trip at the company's expense."

"I was going to have lunch with Andrew tomorrow," Brian objected.

"This isn't a request, Craig," Wright growled. "Naylor is deadly serious. The whole business doesn't smell right to him, either. He suspects foul play at a high level." He leant over and picked up a piece of paper from his desk and handed it to Brian. "Flight leaves at six a.m. from the domestic terminal. Put the heavies on this Travers character. Southport is expecting you. Don't run up any fancy lunches at the casino or it comes out of your pay."

＊ ＊ ＊

Brian Craig drove his hire car to Southport Hospital at half past nine the next morning. It had been a bumpy flight, plus an hour's delay at Mascot domestic. On arrival at the Gold Coast there had been an unpleasant altercation with the hire car company, who apparently had no record of his booking the night before. These mounting annoyances had compounded to put him into a particularly foul mood. He went straight up to Travers' office and banged on the door. A voice from inside bade him enter with the same tone as Daniel might have been ordered into the lion's den. Brian stepped inside.

"What do you want?" Travers barked. "I'm operating this morning. Do you have an appointment?"

"No." Brian shut the door behind him loudly. "You lodged a complaint concerning a Mr. James, reporter from Sydney."

"What if I did?" Travers scowled. "Who the devil are you?"

"Detective from Sydney. What exactly was this Mr. James interested in?"

"I have nothing further to say." Travers began to get out of his chair. "If you want to know what I told him, ask him."

"Doctor Travers," Brian said curtly, "we can conduct this interview in this room or down at Southport police station, where it will be more formal and much less pleasant. Take your pick." He dragged a chair towards Travers' desk and sat down. "Oh, and I don't give a damn about your operating schedule."

Brian thought Travers was going to explode. Slowly, as he watched, reason took the place of seething rage. With an expression of sheer dislike, Travers threw the folder he was holding down on his desk. With a sigh of resignation, he sat back down in his chair and half closed his eyes.

"And they say the police are here to help us," he muttered. "James came here to ask about a patient, a girl with severe neurological damage – caused by electrocution, I think. She was in a coma, and if she ever came out of it she would have been severely impaired, hardly able to function at all." He grimaced. "Her mother was one of those dreadful specimens who are allergic to self-sacrifice and wasn't coping with the situation. She had some playboy type hanging around her in the beginning, but he soon shuffled off for greener pastures. A more self-serving, self-pitying specimen of the human race would be hard to find."

"The girl died?" Brian asked.

"Yes, but I have my suspicions." Travers grimaced again. "The whole incident was bizarre. Some doctor – the reporter mentioned his name, Ferris, from Sydney, was on the ward that night, why I don't know, and he apparently pronounced her dead sometime in the morning. When I arrived her body was already on its way to Sydney for cremation."

"Your suspicions?" Brian extracted a notebook from his pocket.

"I think the woman may have hired him to murder her child. As I said, she was a completely self-serving specimen with no thought for her own daughter. I've no doubt the child was dead when she left. What worries me is how she might have died."

"You voiced these suspicions to anyone?" Brian asked, scribbling in his notebook.

"Apart from you, no," Travers frowned heavily. "I lodged a complaint with hospital management and never heard a thing from them. I'm a busy man, detective. Who did you say you were?"

"Craig. What was the child's name?"

"I can't remember. I was so boiling mad I took the girl's files down to administration and told them I washed my hands of the whole incident. Didn't want any repercussions coming in my direction. Guess that was a bit naïve."

"You have absolutely no idea who the girl was, even after you treated her for how long?" Brian asked incredulously.

"Several weeks." Travers picked up the folder on his desk, indicating by the expression on his face that the interview was fast coming to an end. "No. Detective Craig, since that night over four years ago, I have treated around seven hundred patients. Do you expect me to remember all their names? Normally I keep files. In this case, no. I've explained why."

"The administration could tell me, then. Surely they would have had admission records."

"You don't keep up with what's going on in your own country, do you?" Travers said sarcastically.

"What d'you mean?" Brian retorted.

"Remember what happened around November last year? I thought every Australian would remember that. I suppose if it happens in some other state you Cockroaches from down south don't give a damn."

"There was a cyclone, wasn't there?" Brian said, wrinkling his forehead. "I know there was a lot of flooding in Brisbane. Did you get flooded down here too?"

"Did we get flooded," Travers grunted. "The whole ground floor was half under water. Most hospital records were lost forever."

"Surely they would have had some sort of backup," Brian asked.

"I don't know." He stood up. "Go ask them, incompetent lot of little paper pushers that they are."

Brian thanked Travers for his help, wished him a pleasant morning operating, and walked the short distance to the Admissions and Administration building. By the time he left he felt so sympathetic towards Travers he thought he might even go back to his office and tell him so. Glancing at his watch, he realised the good doctor would be in theatre and decided to leave matters lie. No one in administration could tell him anything about the incident. Not only couldn't they, it took a long phone call to Southport police station before they would believe who he was. When they realised he had been telling them the truth, they began to duck shove all responsibility onto the shoulders of those unfortunately not able to be present through transfer, retirement or death. The General Manager was called, a gentleman in his early forties who looked sixty something. He had a nervous twitch, and a habit of repeating the phrase 'you know' over and over again.

"An act of God, you know, that flood, terrible, people lost their lives, you know. Doctor Travers is responsible for keeping his own records, you know. We sent him a memo, so if the records have been lost it's his own damn fault, you know."

Brian caught the four o'clock plane back to Sydney after a pleasant lunch at a Southport pub. The next morning he gave Wright his only two pieces of information. There was a dead girl who could have been murdered, and there was a doctor Ferris who could be followed up.

Wright fiddled around a bit with the computer on his desk. He sent some stuff to the printer and grimaced. "Doctor David Ferris, neurologist, lecturer at Sydney University faculty of medicine, working at Westmead in some research group, was found dead in the Parramatta river two days after the storm." He handed Brian the printed sheet. "You remember the storm, Craig?"

"I remember the storm."

"You didn't waste your time up in Queensland. There has to be a connection with the Storm girl. This Ferris worked at Westmead, close to where you picked her up. Find out what Ferris was working on, Craig. More importantly, who he was working with. Not much to go on is it? You're sure no one had any idea who the girl was?"

Brian took the sheet of paper. "They were all dodging for cover. Seems as though everyone was too busy shifting patients or getting themselves into boats to worry about their computer systems on the night of the flood."

Over the next week Brian made several trips to the medical research unit at Westmead. Each time he was told something different. No Doctor Ferris had ever worked there. No, they couldn't tell him the name of any project or the names of his colleagues because they had no record that he had ever worked there. Perhaps he could contact the University of Sydney directly.

Every enquiry in that direction had met the same bureaucratic confusion. Nobody knew anything about a project running at Westmead campus. The research centre had yet to be completed. They were waiting for new equipment. No, they didn't have the details on hand.

Wright conveyed their frustration to the Commissioner in expressive if restrained language. All he could tell Brian, was that the Commissioner's interest in the case had intensified greatly.

Chapter 24

Frankfurt, same year

Outside the window a freezing rain sleeted down. The black sky threatened to send further violent offerings against the thin glass which rattled in its loose fitting frame. A few unfortunate citizens hurried past, their covered heads bowed against the elements, their sodden feet splashing on the cobbles awash with icy water. Inside the room it had grown dark, too dark to conduct further business. Gerhardt Metzger turned on the meagre light and shut the curtains against the miserable scene, pausing to glance at his BMW parked against the kerb, the rain sheeting off its dark blue roof. A labour, hardly of love, mostly of duty, this monotonous disposal of Tante Frieda's simple earthly possessions. Most of them had already turned to ash in the fireplace which heated the room. The flickering flame cast shadows on the faded plaster walls, yellowed with age, now dying down as the last armful of paper had been consumed. At least he was warm.

He paused briefly to examine the portrait hanging on the wall in its modern glassless frame, the portrait drawn by some young woman in Australia. Yes, it was a good likeness. He reached up and took it down. A few blows with his foot reduced the frame to kindling and the drawing to torn paper. He threw them into the fire. He opened the roll top desk. Yes, it was in good condition, and would fetch a few euros in the Frankfurt antique markets. He began to open the drawers and tip their contents directly into the fire without even looking at them. How demeaning, he thought, to reach the end of one's life with nothing more than a few handfuls of paper to show you had ever been.

The last bundle fell into the fire, all save a small newspaper cutting. He picked it up and was about to throw it into the rising flames when he stopped, stared at the image and took it over to where the light was stronger, holding it up towards the glimmering bulb. All thought of disposal forgotten, he walked over to the ancient leather lounge and sat down, the scrap of paper still clenched in his hand. Life, he pondered, had taken some strange twists and turns, but none stranger than this. For a long time he sat there staring into the dying flames. Then, pausing only to turn out the light, he shouldered his greatcoat, donned his cap and scarf and went out into the storm. Inside the car he removed his soaking garments leaving only shirt and trousers. He grabbed a thick woollen jumper from the back seat and put it on, started the engine and waited until the impenetrable fog had cleared from the windscreen. It was a slow journey back to his quarters inside the Goethe-Universität, the sheeting rain reducing visibility to near zero at times. He was thankful so few other vehicles were braving the difficult conditions, thankful the Führungskräfte Unterkünfte had underground parking with lift access to his rooms.

Ten minutes later he was typing 'Ellen Craig' into his desktop computer. There was only one entry, an Ellen Craig, thirteen years old, only daughter of Drs. A & B Craig of Cherrybrook NSW Australia, close to where the teenage artist had wielded her trade. Coincidence? Metzger was not a believer in coincidences. Yet how was this possible? The girl had almost certainly been cremated, and Ferris was dead, possibly at the hands of his brother in law's shady friends. But what if the impossible had happened? Her soul had somehow come to life and she had been resurrected? What utter nonsense, what fantasy. He reproved himself severely. This was the sort of rubbish that had fragmented the group towards the end, some tacit adherence to a metaphysical reality, even while they vociferously denied it.

Yet what if it was?

In that case there was a family called Craig who were protecting her, a family who didn't know her real name, and were willing to lend her one of theirs. The implications were staggering. For the second time in a minute he found himself appealing to that same metaphysical reality for explanation, the same superstitious nonsense he had spent his life refuting. People did not rise from the dead. There was some other explanation, however improbable. She was a doppelganger. Occam's razor, the simplest explanation was probably the correct one. But what if, for whatever reason, tissue library twenty nine was still available to complete their research so prematurely cut short?

It would have to be re-acquired and rendered incapable of further resurrection. Amputation of its limbs, perhaps. Yes, a simple surgical process, and perhaps several others which would ensure no further surprises were possible. No, surely this could not have happened, but he would find out. There was work to be done. All at once the prospect of reaching his frustrated goal loomed large before his eyes. This time science would not be blended with sentimentality, and he would die knowing his existence would be remembered for far more than a desk full of useless paper.

Come to think of it, not quite useless. There was work to be done.

CHAPTER 25

Hunt shoved the Visa card into the machine and nodded at the truckie across the counter. "Pump number eight, three sausage rolls and the magazine. Credit or savings account, Sir?"

"Credit and make it quick, mate," the truckie said with a weary voice.

Hunt made it quick. He smiled as he thought of the truckie trying to eat three sausage rolls which had been steadily petrifying on the heating rack all day. Perhaps he wouldn't notice, absorbed in his latest edition of sleaze, sold inside an opaque wrapping with a large black 'R restricted' on the front. Why the garage stocked the rubbish he couldn't imagine, not many people bought it. He glanced at his watch, three a.m. What a job. He surveyed the brightly illuminated concrete apron in front of the petrol station. No customers in sight. In an hour or two they would come rolling in, sleepy eyed, cross and suffering from caffeine withdrawal as they began their daily commute. Right now he could concentrate on other matters.

Reaching down, he hauled his briefcase up onto the counter and opened it. This investigation was enough to make him wish he had never chosen journalism as a career. He flipped through the first dozen profiles of everyone on the list he had covertly obtained from the medical research centre, photographs, biographies, credentials. He would recognise any of them by sight if they walked into the garage, yet not one of them had he been able to interview. Since the night of the storm they had scattered like rats leaving a sinking ship. Metzger had returned to Germany, Hargraves and Ross were working for some pharmaceutical company in the States, Yanac in Amsterdam, Festerhaus untraceable, Ferris, dead. Krishna, the physiotherapist, could have been in the same condition for all he knew. Brown was such a common name he hadn't even bothered to try, and Cornish had vanished off the face of the planet. His last name, Lucknow, may have gone to Germany with Metzger, but he had received no answer to several emails sent to Goethe-Universität. All in all a complete dead end.

There was but one lead he hadn't followed. Ferris had a younger sister who had married. If he could trace her name... He opened the web browser on the garage computer terminal. Just before the first bleary eyed customer walked into the garage at four twenty a.m. he thought he might have it, Joan Burgess nee Ferris, married to a Fred Burgess, a manager out at Northern Suburbs crematorium, right age, living in Eastwood, not all that far away. A few hours' sleep and he would pay her a visit. His shift was due to end at eight a.m.

Joan Burgess was obviously employed somewhere during the day since no one was picking up on their home number. Hunt had to wait a couple of days until his shift at the garage changed before he could see her the following Thursday evening.

Hunt walked up to the large brass security gate enclosing the complex of luxury townhouses on Blaxland road and pushed the button marked 'Eight'.

A woman's voice answered. "Yes? Who are you?"

The words were pitched slightly high, and sounded agitated. Care was obviously called for.

"This is a Mr. James, Mrs Burgess. I'm a freelance reporter writing an article on the incredible work done by your brother, Doctor David Ferris prior to his tragic death. I'm trying to obtain some personal information to make his character a little more accessible to those who will read about him. I was wondering if you could assist me."

"I … don't think so… It's good of you, but…" The woman's voice wavered with uncertainty.

"Your brother was a great man, Mrs. Burgess," Hunt continued with all the feigned sincerity he could muster. "From my research I believe he was quite brilliant, yet he has disappeared into obscurity without so much as a mention. I would seek to redress that injustice, Mrs. Burgess."

"I suppose… when will this article be published? In what paper?" Mrs. Burgess said nervously.

"A couple of reputable medical journals are interested. I can't give you their names I'm afraid, and there is a possibility the Australian will carry the story."

"I'm not sure I can be of much assistance Mr. James. Come on up."

There was a click and the door unlatched. Hunt whisked himself through and made his way across the paved courtyard, past the expensive fountains and exquisitely manicured gardens to the town house at the end, number eight. He knocked on the large mahogany door. A slight woman with mousey brown hair, hazel eyes and a worried expression on her somewhat angular face opened the door and beckoned him inside.

"Fred is a little late this evening," she stammered. "I hope he's not going to mind. Now, Mr. James, can I get you a coffee?"

"No, thanks. Could you tell me, as his sister, what did you think of his research?"

"His research?" Mrs. Burgess replied nervously. "With that pharmaceutical company? He wouldn't talk about it."

"No, his research with the University," Hunt prompted.

"I don't know anything about that." She frowned deeply. "David was working for a pharmaceutical company until the day he died. I know, because they gave us quite a lot of compensation."

248

"At Westmead campus?"

"Yes, along with dear Professor Isaac. Such a gentleman."

"And what pharmaceutical company was that, Mrs—"

At that instant the door opened, and a large man with black hair and eyebrows to match strode into the room. He stared at Hunt then his wife, his face like thunder. Mrs. Burgess appeared to shrink into the shag pile carpet.

"Who is this turd, Joan? What's he doing here?" the man bellowed.

"This is Mr. James," Mrs. Burgess quavered. "He's writing an article on David."

"Get out!" Burgess' eyes blazed.

Hunt recognised the look. It usually preceded a punch up, and by the size of the man and the expression on his face, there was no guarantee the altercation would go in Hunt's preferred direction, which was Hunt uninjured and his opponent lying unconscious on the floor. He made one attempt to recover the situation.

"Your wife was happy to have me collect some information about her brother, a brilliant man who deserves—"

"What part of 'get out' can't a dumb assed reporter understand?" the man growled.

He put down his briefcase and began to take off his coat. Not good signs. He was standing to the left of the front door in the short hallway which separated the living room from the entrance, waiting for his unwelcome visitor to walk past so he could administer a little reminder not to pay a second visit. Mrs. Burgess continued to sink into the carpet, her hands shaking visibly.

Hunt selected a tone of nervous compliance. "I... I'm sorry Mr. Burgess. I'm sure there is no need for unpleasantness. I regret disturbing your wife. I'll be going now."

He moved towards the door, tensed like a spring, still maintaining his demeanour of frightened subservience. Burgess was now close to his left shoulder. Out of the corner of his eye he saw the movement, the rising knee going for his shin. Burgess, just for a second, was standing on one foot. In a lightning move Hunt stepped back, grabbed him by the neck and shoved his head through the plaster wall on the other side of the hall. So great was the force of the shove that Burgess' head went right through into the room beyond. Mrs. Burgess screamed, but Hunt paid no attention. The man was a crim if ever he saw one, no doubt with a number of unpleasant colleagues who would be causing Hunt further trouble unless he made his point. Before Burgess could get his head out of the hole he kicked him hard in the stomach. As he jerked back through the wall, Hunt delivered a smashing blow to his jaw which threw him against the opposite wall. Another blow to his stomach and Burgess went down in a heap, demolishing the delicate hat stand beside the door.

"Now Burgess," Hunt said, breathing hard, "I'm leaving like you wanted. If any unpleasant present arrives in the future, I will assume it's from you, and my Fed mates will be crawling all over your little world like ants on a dead rat. Understand?"

The figure on the carpet made a slight nodding movement with his blood and plaster covered head. Hunt walked through the door and closed it after him. *That poor woman is going to have a very bad night,* he thought, *the price you paid for marrying scum.* The man was a crim alright, conveniently working at the crematorium. He shuddered to think of the implications. Another dead end.

Back in his home at Cherrybrook he put some antiseptic cream on his skinned knuckles, and taking a beer out of the fridge opened the folder from his briefcase. All the academics were missing or accounted for. Two of the three physiotherapists had vanished into thin air, and the other had the ubiquitous name of Brown. Hopeless. Cornish was the lead to follow, if there was any lead left to follow.

Four days later he had a breakthrough. A Patricia Cornish had married a Tony Fletcher six years ago, now living in Gosford on the Central Coast. A search under the name of Patricia Fletcher came up with a physiotherapy clinic in the same suburb, enough of a coincidence to make the two hour drive worthwhile. Another week passed before he could take a break from the garage, then driving with the help of his GPS, he arrived at the pleasant cream brick house in Maiden's Brush Road and rang the bell.

A man, presumably Tony Fletcher, answered, and reluctantly led him into the lounge room where he found Patricia Fletcher looking nervous. Hunt concocted some plausible story about preparing an article on the life and work of Doctor Isaac Gilead, which they clearly didn't believe. The mention of Gilead's name did not produce the same reaction as it had in Mrs. Burgess. He noticed Tony's fist clench involuntarily, and read the fear in his wife's rather lovely blue eyes.

"I'm afraid I can't help you, Mr. James," Patricia Fletcher stammered. "You see, I joined the research group because the money was fantastic, and it was supposed to be a long term proposition. Tony worked with a computer firm in Sydney then, and it was so convenient. We rented at Northmead. The project didn't last as long as expected. They made us all sign a confidentiality agreement when we started, and another when we left. If I break it I'm in really big trouble."

From the fear on her attractive face Hunt believed it.

"Can you tell me, was the work done for the University of Sydney, or some pharmaceutical company?" Hunt said in his most persuasive voice.

The young woman gazed appealingly towards her husband. He came over to stand beside her. He was afraid too, Hunt thought.

"I believe the University rented us the rooms, Mr. James, that's all I can say," she stammered. "I'm not allowed to name the company. Please understand. We would like to help. It was a mistake, a terrible mistake."

There were tears in her eyes now as well as fear. His initial suspicions were correct. No university would implement the level of security he had seen at Westmead. No university would be so damn cagey. Publicity attracted research dollars, and whoever was running the Westmead group wanted neither. Shock tactics were called for.

"Mrs. Fletcher, I'm sorry to distress you. I'm actually investigating what could be a connection between the project you were working on and organised crime."

"Mercy!" The blue eyes were wide with fear now. Tony Fletcher put his arm protectively around her shoulders.

"I'm afraid I have to ask you to leave, Mr. James," he said firmly. "You're distressing my wife."

"I promise to go if you will answer this last question," Hunt said as gently as he could. "I also promise not to reveal the source of this information to anyone. What were three physiotherapists doing in a neurological research project?"

"We were taking care of a patient who needed constant attention," Mrs. Fletcher stammered. "Please, Mr. James, we want to put the whole thing behind us. I'm sorry I ever became involved. It was the money. I was a fool to agree, but I did. Please honour your promise. We just want to be left alone to raise a family and do what we can to help people."

"I believe you. Thank you Mr. and Mrs. Fletcher. If you ever wish to contact me—" Hunt took a card out of his pocket with his alias and a mobile phone number. He handed it to the husband who nearly snatched it out of his hand.

He drove back to Sydney in a thoughtful mood.

So the plot had thickened considerably. No wonder he had found the University uncooperative when he had contacted the Dean of the faculty. They had hired out their space to someone else, probably for a handsome sum which no doubt paid the bill for other projects, yet the space on the Westmead campus had not reverted to University use. Now that was strange. Was the venerable Doctor Ferris engaged in criminal activity as well as his brother-in-law? Something had to explain the project's collapse the day he died. Next he had to discover the name of the company involved or the project they were working on. Whatever it was, there was plenty of money and clout involved. Perhaps they stood to make a fortune from their clandestine research. That would account for the reaction of the Fletchers. Some pharmaceutical companies paid millions for the latest medical research, which they would recoup a thousand fold in drug sales.

CHAPTER 26

The stranger approached Storm with a look in his eyes which she had learned to recognise. A whole term had passed so quickly, she had learnt so much, both from the social environment as well as her lecturers. The young man spotted the crutches beside her chair and frowned. *Didn't expect that, did you?* Storm thought to herself. *Now you're pretending to read messages on your phone so you don't have to talk to the hot chick who's lame. There's plenty of girls down the other end of the canteen, all from Fashion. You can tell by the way they're dressed. Take your pick.* She laughed to herself as the young man retreated in her predicted direction.

She opened her backpack and fished out some sandwiches to eat with the cup of coffee she had bought a few minutes ago, and smiled quietly to herself. Crutches were such an unexpected asset at Sydney Institute. For starters they kept the predatory males off, and there were quite a few of those, but they also seemed to confer a certain privileged status upon her amongst the staff and management. Nearly every day someone would come into the classroom and ask her how she was coping. Was there was anything else they could do to make her life as a disabled student easier? Did she have trouble getting into the lifts, did she have any difficulty negotiating the access ramps, did she need counselling to help with her self-esteem? No, she didn't. She had conveyed this simple message a hundred times before, but they kept on coming nonetheless.

It had taken her a few weeks to recognise three distinct groups of students in her course. There were those who came because they had a friend, usually of the opposite sex, who was doing the course with them. These paid little attention to what was going on about them, and usually disappeared around assignment time. Then there were those who came because they were paid to be there by the government study assistance scheme, and it was easy money. All they had to do was attend class, which most of them did, sitting up the back, bored or stoned or both. Some of the third group came to have another go at the Higher School Certificate which they had already sat for in school the previous year.

The remainder were from various sorts of educationally disadvantaged backgrounds who were doing their best with the extra chance this excellent institute provided them. There was a considerable range of ability within these, and Storm soon discovered she was the leader of the pack. It was a nice feeling getting the highest marks in every assignment, but although she could rest on her laurels and still top the class, it didn't necessarily mean she would do very well against all the other students in the state, some of whom came from prestigious high schools.

Studying carefully the way the marks were calculated and moderated between schools, she worked out there was only one thing to be done. She had to top her course in every subject, top the institute, and do well enough to compete against these other gifted students in the external exam. Her lecturers, once they heard of her ambition, proved incredibly helpful and enthusiastic. They gave her extra work. They spent hours in private tutorials in their own time. Somehow they managed to obtain copies of tests and assignments from a number of those prestigious schools and set her to work on them, marking her hard and then showing her how to improve. In fact, although she had no inkling of it, 'Helen Craig for Medicine' had become the goal of the faculty. The staff who taught her would meet weekly to monitor her progress and plan ways to improve it. A student of this calibre, from such an educationally disadvantaged and tantalisingly obscure background, represented both an unparalleled opportunity and a unique challenge to bring glory and honour to the faculty. Besides, she was a delightful young woman, and they had all become quite fond of her.

Storm finished her sandwich, fished out her Bible, and began to read where she left off that morning. A Bible was also a useful deterrent. Most people left her alone when she began to read it. Occasionally someone would make a disparaging comment as they walked past, but she had learned to ignore them. Once or twice she had discovered another follower of the Way, which was nice, and they had become friends. The prevailing attitude amongst the students was do your own thing and let others do theirs. So she wanted to read the Bible, well that was okay, as long as she didn't try to pour all that religious nonsense over anyone else.

Being the top student brought its own share of problems. None of her fellow students in any of her classes failed to recognise her academic ability. Several of the more unscrupulous had tried to take advantage of it by getting her to do problems in their assignments. Storm had refused, somewhat lessening her popularity but not her reputation. Others, such as Kim Nguyen who was fast approaching the table, had unashamedly asked for help. Despite warnings from all her teachers that she shouldn't waste her precious study time helping lame puppies, Storm often did precisely that.

Kim came over, gave Storm a quick sisterly embrace and sat down. "I can't do number four in the maths," she said, "can you do if for me?"

"No," Storm said, smiling, "but I'll teach you how, okay?"

"You're so cool. Want some of my orange juice?"

Storm put her Bible back into her backpack. Paul's letter to the Romans required concentration, and would have to wait. Fifteen minutes of explanation followed.

"How come you're so bright?" Kim said, packing her folder back into her bag. "It's so easy when you explain it. George Tanner showed us this morning and I didn't have a clue what he was talking about."

"God's gift, Kim. George is a bit obscure at times. I have a brother, Peter, who showed me that trick last year, so you see I'm not all that clever."

"I've never heard of anyone who believes in God like you. You're always singing quietly about it in Biology practicals. Must make you really happy."

"You want to have a singing heart too, Kim?"

"I gotta go and see Khine over there," Kim said hastily. "She's got my English assignment. Thanks for the help. Ciao."

That was a fairly typical response whenever Storm offered to talk about following the Way. She glanced up surprised. The young man who had walked past her before was back and making his way directly over to her table.

"Hi," he said. "Sorry to walk past you before. I had to see a mate down the other end of the canteen. What course are you doing here?"

"Higher School Certificate," Storm answered.

"Great to have a second chance, isn't it?" He sat down at the table uninvited. "Did the same thing year before last. Second year Electrical Engineering now. Fooled around a bit at school, then did a hairdressing course."

"You didn't like being a hairdresser?" Storm began to shoulder her back pack. There was something about the stranger she didn't like.

"Actually I did,' he continued in a friendly manner, "but I thought it was a bit of a dead loss job. You've got really lovely hair, did you know that?"

"No." Storm clipped her shoulder strap shut.

"I used to have this speciality. Lots of young women went for it. I'd lift their hair up – do you mind? Like this."

He reached over and lifted Storm's hair up high on her head.

"Then I'd curl it on top of your head like—"

Storm pushed his hand away. "Please don't touch my hair, I don't like it when strangers touch my hair."

"Sorry. Just wanted to show you, no offence meant."

"What did you say your name was?" Storm asked.

"Tony Wilson. And you are?"

"Helen. I have to go now, Tony. 'Bye."

She stood up, fixed her arms in her crutches and made her way out of the canteen as quickly as possible. Something wasn't right. As soon as he had lifted her hair she had felt goose bumps up and down her arms. A truly awful thought struck her. Abandoning her afternoon English lecture for the first time, she made her way down to Enrolments and Course Information. Assembling her face into exactly the right sad, worried expression she went up to the counter.

"I hope you can help me," she stammered. "My name's Emma Wilson, and I'm searching for my brother who is enrolled in Electrical Engineering. We're from South Australia and our Mum is very, very ill, not going to live much longer." She squeezed a tear out of her eye. "I have to find him. He left home very badly three years ago, and I've only just traced him here – or I think it's here. I know there are other Institutes. Could you please tell me if there's a Tony Wilson enrolled in second year Electrical Engineering?"

"I'm sorry, Miss Wilson, we're not supposed to divulge this information." The girl behind the counter said stiffly.

"Please." More tears. "I won't ask anything else. I'll go and see the Head Teachers and ask them, but it's such a waste if he's not at this Institute. I haven't a lot of time left, and Mum really wants to see her... her son before she... she..."

Storm pulled out a large handkerchief from her bag and covered her face with it. Ellen would be proud of her. She felt absolutely dreadful for lying, but she had to find out. She made to turn away from the counter, but the girl on the other side spoke suddenly.

"Don't go just yet, Miss Wilson. I'll tell you if there's someone of that name enrolled and then it's up to you to go to Electrical Engineering and see if you can locate him. It must be awful for you, disabled and all. Wait a moment." She spent a minute or two typing into the computer terminal on the counter. "Wilson? No, there's no Tony Wilson enrolled here. Are you all right, Miss Wilson? Would you like some help getting down the access ramp?"

Storm's face had suddenly turned very pale. "That's really disappointing. I was hoping... I'll have to go somewhere else," she stammered.

"It could have been the University of Technology. That was once called an Institute. You could try there. I'm searching all Institute enrolments now, and there's no T. Wilson in any year of Electrical Engineering."

Storm thanked her and went back to her class, unable to concentrate on anything. Perhaps she was worrying about nothing. The young man could have easily given her a false name after she had brushed him off for touching her hair. Yes, that was probably what had happened. Boys acted really stupid when they felt rejected. "Come on, Storm," she said to herself, "this isn't like you to worry about nothing. I'm a follower of Jesus, and He's taking care of me. What a storm in a teacup." She laughed quietly at her own joke and felt a bit better. *Concentrate, Storm. You won't remain top of the class if you keep this up,* she thought to herself, but deep down inside her fear remained. Somehow the darkness was reaching out for her, and despite her attempts at denial, she knew it.

Peter Craig had gone to bed that night with a headache. Human anatomy required a superhuman memory. He was always forgetting small details, the same small details his lecturers, by some foul sixth sense, knew he had forgotten. Then they could ask him embarrassing questions about them and turn him into the village idiot, just as they had today. He had shut the textbook as the words were starting to run together. Beyond this point he would begin to unlearn all the stuff he had crammed into his brain over the previous three hours. Soon after his head touched the pillow he was asleep.

It was the scream which woke him up, followed by another one.

He heard feet running down the hall past his bedroom door. He vaulted out of bed and shot into the hallway, trying to collect his wits. There was a light in his parent's room and another in Storm's. Instinctively he ran towards the latter and burst in to find Basa sitting up on the bed. Storm's head was buried in her breast, and she was sobbing her heart out. Her arms were wrapped around his mother and she was shaking like a leaf.

"What's happened?" he asked breathlessly.

"It's alright, Peter." Basa turned towards her son in the doorway. "Storm had a really bad dream. She's fine now, but I'm going to stay with her for a while. Go to bed, Peter, Storm's alright. Go back to bed, *now*." Basa laid emphasis on the last word.

He saw Storm nod her head without lifting it from its comforting place. He turned round and went back to his own bedroom, shutting the door behind him. Why did he feel so annoyed? Storm was in the very best of hands. Mum would stay with her all night if needs be, until whatever it was had passed. He had a wonderful, caring Mum and he thanked God for her. Why was he feeling so inexplicably resentful? Tired, he must be tired. He lay there in the dark recalling the image of Storm's face buried in his mother's breast, and suddenly knew what was bothering him.

He wanted to be the one to comfort her.

He wanted her head on his own chest, his own arms around her. He was the one to protect her, and he had been shut out, not through jealousy,

260

but by his own mother's careful understanding. She was right. Storm was frightened and vulnerable. He was the knight in shining armour come to hold the damsel in his arms, and he knew his caring brother act would be stretched to the limit considering the bedroom environment.

He had come to hate the role, but it was the only one which kept him in Storm's world, and he knew he could live in no other place. She was his but not his, there but not there, close but not close enough. Storm's heart was as pure as the driven snow. He was her brother, and she loved him. He would have to be content with that. If he told her the truth he would lose her, destroy all the beautiful expressions of innocent intimacy which he craved for, the joy in her eyes, the laughter in her voice, the singing. Life would be over the day he lost them. But one day he would. The beautiful creature would spread her wings and find she could fly.

He groaned audibly and turned over and tried to go to sleep. Despite his tiredness, sleep would not come. Storm's only other nightmare was after Harris had tried it on, so what had sponsored this one? Something at the Institute, that was it. He would find out, oh yes he would. He might not be able to hold her in his arms on her bed, but he wouldn't stand by while some other male predator advanced on the woman he loved. *Maybe I'll take a day or two off from Medicine and come with her*, he thought, and then no one would find out about those little pieces of anatomy he couldn't remember. Pity help anyone who made the slightest move towards her then. He mightn't be the best fighter around, but determination made up for a great deal. The picture pleased him. Some male creep lying on the floor bleeding, and Storm's body pressed against his, whispering her love and desire in his ear. Much better. With this delightful scene spread out before his imagination he drifted off to sleep.

❋ ❋ ❋

The next day began better than his wildest dreams. It wasn't yet five a.m. The grey light of dawn barely penetrated the heavy bedroom curtains. He was suddenly awakened by a soft knocking at his door, and then a dressing-gowned figure was kneeling at the side of his bed, her arms around his shoulders, dragging him towards her.

"Peter, I know what you felt last night," Storm whispered softy. "I didn't need to see. Hold me."

Peter reached out his arms and held her. How could she have known? He felt her kisses on his cheek, the scent of her hair falling all over his face, her soft breath warm on his neck. For an insane second he wondered if she too might have been disappointed, might have wished for what he had so passionately desired.

"You will always be my protector, Peter," Storm assured him. "No one else, no one ever. Mum is very wise, Peter. She understands both of us better than you know. You were hurt. Please don't be hurt, Peter. I ache inside when you're hurt."

He was nearly at the point of telling her, but no, the risk was too great. This was a beautiful moment, and nothing in the world was going to cast a shadow over it. He wrapped his arms around her shoulders and held her tightly against him.

"It was the darkness, Peter," she confided in an unsteady voice. "Something happened yesterday. It was a silly, trivial thing, but I suddenly went cold, as though some dark and evil arm had stretched out long, long, and found me. I thought I had forgotten all about it, then I had this dream – it was horrible."

Her arms tightened ferociously around his shoulders. Peter slipped out from under the covers and sat on the side of the bed, folding his arms around her back and holding her close against him. She was shaking all over again.

"I was lying down on something. I hated being there but I couldn't move, couldn't – wake up, that was it. Then this man came, and I knew he was going to kill me. Somehow I was moving down this corridor. There were lights passing above me, and I knew I was going to die when I got to the end. Suddenly it all went black. I thought he'd killed me." She shuddered suddenly.

262

STORM DANCING

"There was this terrible crash, and I was flying out of control through the darkness. All of a sudden I smashed into something, and then I'm on the ground. I can't see, but I'm awake. I can move my arms and legs. I know the man is coming to kill me and I'm terrified, because I can't find a way out. I bash into this solid thing and there's a lever in my hand. I push on it and it's raining. I suddenly feel better. Then these lights blaze out in the dark and I scream. I woke up then. I think I screamed too, because the next second Mum is holding me. Hold me, Peter. Hold me tight, please."

Peter drew her against him. He kissed her hair, rubbing his face amongst its fragrance, waiting until the shaking began to diminish, felt her breath coming more slowly, deeper.

"You've told Mum all this?" he whispered tenderly.

"Uh-huh."

"What does she think?"

"She thinks I'm remembering something that happened just before uncle Brian rescued me from that drain thing. She's a bit worried about what happened yesterday too, and she's going to tell uncle Brian about it."

"What happened yesterday?" Peter asked, his voice full of concern.

"Some stranger who said he was a hairdresser lifted my hair up. I didn't like it. I asked his name, then I found out he'd lied to me. Silly, isn't it?"

"No it isn't silly," Peter said with conviction. "I'm coming to the Institute with you today. Nothing happens to you while I'm alive."

"Peter, you have lectures," Storm protested quietly. "I'm not letting my stupid fears interfere with your study."

"Storm, how do you think I'd feel if anything happened to you?" Peter said, emotion surging through his voice. "My life would end, Storm. Don't you know that?"

"Dearest Peter." She turned and kissed him tenderly on the cheek. "I've become such a burden, haven't I? I really should go."

At least five more minutes passed before she acted on her own advice. Even then it was obvious to Peter she didn't want to leave him. He got out of bed, wrapped his dressing gown around him, and taking her hand, went out into the breakfast room. Basa was already there. The frown said it all.

"I went in to see Peter this morning, Mum," Storm explained. "I'm sorry. I haven't been there very long. It wasn't Peter's fault. He wants to go to the Institute with me today. I told him I was just being silly."

"I've phoned uncle Brian." Basa said matter-of-factly.

"What?" Peter said. "At five a.m.?"

"He's on a night shift. I phoned him last night after Storm had gone to sleep. He's coming with you today, not Peter, and he's clearing it with the Institute management. Don't worry, you mightn't even see him, but there'll be someone keeping an eye on things. You should have trusted me a little more, Storm. We talked about that."

Storm looked so woebegone it made Basa laugh.

"No damage done. Yes, Peter, uncle Brian is concerned too, but you needn't worry someone will take Storm away. Set the table, will you? Ellen's sleeping in late again. Must speak sternly to that girl."

Peter set the table. Still the sensation of Storm's embrace and her kisses lingered in his mind. There was no escaping the truth. He was desperately in love with her. Only in that brief encounter had he dared imagine she could have felt the same way about him. Now his mind repudiated the thought. In her mind he was her brother, her protector, nothing more. That was why she had sought him out. He groaned silently. He was afraid. Before his imagination a dark and evil arm was groping out for her, seeking to possess her and drag her back into the darkness away from him. The worried expression on his face was the only outward sign of the turmoil in his heart.

264

Uncle Brian shadowed Storm for the rest of the week, but nothing unusual happened. The so called Tony Wilson never made an appearance. No other stranger approached her, and by the end of the week he was told to lay off. Storm continued with her studies, and everything returned to normal, or at least the appearance of normality.

Appearances are often deceiving.

CHAPTER 27

Isaac Gilead returned from a less than satisfactory lecture to third year medical students at MIT. He threw his notes down in a pile on his cluttered desk, and slumped down hard into the comfortable leather chair. He had spent four hours preparing that lecture, slides, notes, some practical examples. For all the response he received, he could have spent five minutes, or made it up as he went along. Students these days just sat there, staring vacantly and disinterested. Sometimes he had been tempted to prattle on with complete garbage, just to see how long he could do it before anybody noticed. Perhaps no one would. Even the thought was depressing.

He picked up the latest correspondence from the bioethics committee, opened the envelope, read the contents, screwed it up and hurled it into the wastepaper bin. What did they take him for, a monster? How many good citizens of the USA suffered from dementia, Parkinson's, and other neurological conditions to do with defective structures in the brain? Millions. Here he was, proposing research which would bring relief, which would harm no one, at least no more than they had already been harmed, and every time he was prevented by some form of irrationality. 'Human dignity' was the phrase most often employed, and its incongruity annoyed him intensely. How dignified was a man suffering from dementia? How dignified was a stroke victim, unable to raise food to his mouth? The world was just not ready to embrace the obvious. Perhaps it would remain that way forever.

How he hated religion, the scourge of humanity, from whence came notions of human soul and spirit, notions so fatally confused and useless he marvelled anyone could adhere to them. Life could be so much better if people would simply accept their own organic existence and stop appealing to the heavens for a significance which they already possessed.

The phone rang. Gilead picked it up.

"Hello, am I speaking to Isaac Gilead? Isaac, is that you?"

Gilead almost dropped the instrument in his lap. "Yes, this is Isaac. Gerhardt, is that you? I cannot believe it."

"Es ist gut, deine Stimme, Isaac zu hören. It's me, old friend. How is life treating you in the greater West?"

"I am travelling fairly, Gerhardt, so much better to have heard from you. I believed our relationship to be at an end, both professionally and personally. I must say I have grieved about it. How has life been treating you, my old friend? I trust your family is well. What occasions this call?"

"My aunt died, the rest of the family are well, I am well. Yes, it is good to hear your voice, Isaac. Now I must divulge the purpose of my call. I have discovered a way in which we can complete our research so prematurely cut short by Ferris several years ago."

Gilead could feel his pulse beginning to race, his hand trembled slightly as he pressed the instrument closer to his ear. "You have acquired another tissue library, one with a functioning support system?" he asked softly.

"I received confirmation from Australia only yesterday," Gerhardt said. "Tissue library thirty can be acquired and prepared within a week when all the other laboratory preparations are complete. Remarkable piece of luck, Isaac, I have to say it was, luck."

267

"We can begin work again? There are no bioethical reports to fill in?" Gilead said, breathless with excitement.

"None whatsoever, Isaac," Gerhardt laughed. "I contacted ARG a few days ago, and they are delighted, waiting to hear from you, ready to further their already substantial investment. I assured them there would be no unpleasant repercussions. I will take care of the acquisition of the library and staffing, if you can organise the necessary equipment. How long will it take to refurnish the research centre, do you think?"

"I could do it in six months, Gerhardt. I have a contractual arrangement with MIT which would keep me here until the end of the year, but early next year we could begin. Begin! I am very excited."

"Isaac, Isaac," Gerhardt continued smoothly, "I cannot conceive of accomplishing our goal without you. There are two conditions, however. I am loathe to mention them, but I must."

"These conditions?"

"I am in charge of the team. That is condition one. I am in charge of the tissue library, that is condition two. When we have completed our research, its support system will be shut down, dissected into manageable pieces and incinerated. There will be no attempt made to bring it back to consciousness. Indeed, I don't believe you would consider it. The support system will arrive without limbs, Isaac, so physiotherapy will not be required. Some other superfluous organs may have been removed as well."

"What was it? A motor accident?"

"Don't concern yourself with the details, Isaac, they are all in hand. Perhaps we will be able to overcome the differentiation problem which occurred before. Imagine if we can, when we can. The world will beat a path to our door, Isaac."

"Gerhardt, mein lieber Freund, I would count it an honour to work with you. As for the other, I can see such terrible injuries would preclude any attempt to restore consciousness. Of course I agree."

"I am delighted to hear it, Isaac. There is a third condition which I believe the company will insist on. If you start this project you will stay with it to the end, which will only occur if the support system fails, or we complete our research and shut it down ourselves. I take it you would not object? I believe this will be required in writing prior to any equipment being delivered."

"Yes, yes," Gilead agreed excitedly. "I am not the quitting type, Gerhardt, you know me better than that. I am trembling with anticipation. It has been so frustrating, Gerhardt. I cannot get past the bioethical committees here at all. Every proposal knocked back. I applaud your initiative. Fancy, the team back together again."

"The team will be somewhat different this time, Isaac. I would not employ those physiotherapists, even if we needed them, but our Dr. Lucknow will be useful."

"That man is unbalanced," Gilead objected.

"But brilliant, and we need the MRI images only he can produce. Hargraves, perhaps, not Ross. I will consider Festerhaus if I can find him – it may be difficult with the communists still strutting around in the background. I have some others to approach. Don't worry about staff, Isaac, leave that to me. If you could aim to have the centre humming by early next year it would be perfect."

"I will, I will! Thank you Gerhardt, you have totally changed my mood. I think I was becoming quite depressed. If there is anything else, can you let me know? I will ring our friends in ARG immediately. The paperwork will have to come by special courier. We can't be too careful. I often wonder how Ferris died. Did you learn anything more?"

"Not a thing. He had some very shady connections – useful at the time. When you mix with unscrupulous men you never know quite what they will do."

"There are no unscrupulous men involved this time, I take it, Gerhardt?" Gilead laughed.

"Only me, Isaac. When it comes to our research I am quite without principle. Guten Tag."

Gilead laughed and hung up the phone. Suddenly his head felt light, his heart beat faster. How he had missed the company of his old friend. The project could continue, what an unexpected blessing. He had work to do, lots of work to do, and he would do it with a song in his heart.

CHAPTER 28

I've rung the research centre and told them we're not interested." Ray Wright pulled a large folder from the filing cabinet within arm's reach of his desk.

"We're not?" Brian Craig, sitting opposite, looked incredulous. "What about the lead with Ferris and the dead girl?"

"We're not running the show anymore," Wright said grimly. "Naylor briefed me last night." He picked up the cold coffee from his desk and gulped down the contents, hurling the paper cup into the waste bin. "Apparently Sydney University have no idea who they are renting their own research space to. They damn well know alright, and they aren't going to tell us, and by us I mean the police commissioner's department. You have to have guts to do that, Craig. Big mistake," he grunted.

"Naylor was pretty interested already, now he's like a ferret on acid. He figured out someone must be wielding a pretty big stick to set up bureaucratic countermeasures on that scale, and he wants to know who it is and why. The boys upstairs are busy as beavers."

"So we sit here and do nothing, waiting for the trumpet from on high?" Brian sounded as frustrated as he felt.

"I've been told to lay off, but we're being kept in the loop," Wright said. "Naylor's winkled out an interesting piece of information you'll be pleased to know."

"Yeah? What sort of information?" Brian asked. "Not much use if we're sidelined."

"He's got friends in Australian Border Security, and they've recently had a lot of gear come through for clearance pending delivery to a certain research establishment."

"You don't say," Brian grinned. "Define a lot."

"About thirty five million dollars' worth."

Brian whistled. "Who's splashing that sort of cash around? What sort of gear?"

"One six Tesla MRI machine, latest and greatest, a PET machine, whatever that is, same pedigree, operating theatre type surgical equipment, expensive high-res ultrasound stuff," Wright said, grinning to himself. "There's more, an electron microscope, once again, the best. A FMRI machine, no idea what that does, but it's worth four million itself. Whole lot of other advanced tissue sampling and cryogenic equipment, the sort any hospital ward would give their right arm for."

"And how many beds?" Brian asked. "They must be running a hospital of sorts."

"No beds, but could be local supply. Anyway, the arrival of this stuff has enabled us to breach their security. We know where it's coming from."

"Do tell," Brian said eagerly.

"A big concern in the States, Amity-Rand Genetics. Huge, makes advanced surgical equipment. They control patents on sections of the human genome and some cutting-edge drugs including a new one for prostate cancer. High-end billion dollar show. Pioneered several other medical research programs, one on stem cell harvesting and research."

"Big enough to cover their activities when they don't want others to see," Brian said, nodding his head slowly.

"Plenty big enough to keep prying eyes off commercially sensitive research." Wright leaned forward in his chair. "Whatever they're doing here is bloody important to them Craig, and they don't want people sniffing around watching them do it."

"Any idea what it is?"

"None at all. Neither has Naylor, but he's trying to find out. After the storm everything shut down, and a lot of gear was removed from the place. Most of it was sold to private hospitals and medical imaging centres who could afford the big bikkies. We've only traced some, but so far it's the same sort of gear that's arriving now. Probably planning to continue the same line of research. Why did it stop, why is it starting again?"

"Found a replacement for Ferris, perhaps," Brian suggested.

"Why not just recruit another doctor?" Wright stood up and began pacing the room. "They've got the dough to do it from anywhere in the world. No, I don't think so. Don't forget the boffins skedaddled as well as all the support staff. It was as if a bomb went off in the place. Some internal fricassee which ends in murder? Lots of clever people ducking for cover, no one bleating because they're all too scared."

"Any doves returning to the nest along with this new gear?"

"Not that we know of. The companies who make the gear have sent people to complete its installation. How did we know? They've come through Sydney International, haven't they?"

"Anything you want me to do?" Brian asked enthusiastically.

"Officially, no," Wright grinned. "Unofficially, keep an even closer eye on our superfluous citizen. Naylor's had some academic mates of his search through Australian bioethics proposals submitted over the last ten years, and guess what? This Amity-Rand Genetics hasn't submitted anything."

Wright paused, stared out the window briefly, and then turned to Brian again. "Suppose Ferris wasn't happy, and decides to blow the whole operation to the Australian Bioethics Committee. The storm provides a perfect means of silencing him."

"But what about Storm?" Brian asked. "How does she fit into the picture?"

"Haven't a clue," Wright sighed, "but she's a part of it somehow. Maybe she was delivering pizza or cleaning toilets, when she hears something which could send the rest of them to hell. They grab her and cut the memory out of her brain deliberately. Search me. All I know about medicine is when you're sick, go to a doctor."

"Why not a simple anaesthetic then chuck her into the raging waters?" Brian said thoughtfully. "It was conveniently black as all hell, and by the time they found the body, nobody would even think of testing for suspected murder."

"Don't know, Craig." Wright shook his head. "This whole scenario might be a load of horseshit. Just keep an eye on her, will you? Naylor is going for the company, we can keep tabs on the girl. She's got to be connected somehow."

"Yeah, I'll do that," Brian nodded. "As far as I know no one has shown interest except the non-existent Wilson and our Mr. Hunt. What's he doing by the way?"

"Still working at a garage in Pennant Hills, and avoiding the medical research centre as if they were squirting anthrax into the air."

"Surprised he gave up so easily," Brian mused.

"Don't be too sure about that, Craig. We have to go by the rules, Hunt doesn't. Who knows what little games he's been playing? One day we might have to find out."

Brian grunted at the last comment and walked out of the office. It was almost lunch time and he was starving.

CHAPTER 29

Storm turned over and drew the sheet up tight around her shoulders. Already the early morning light with its summer warmth was streaming brightly through the slit between the bedroom curtains. In the distance she could hear the sounds of morning commuters driving to work. She felt tired. Since the start of the Higher School Certificate exams Basa had insisted she sleep in, and she had, but she had missed the family gathering around the table too. This morning was somehow different. The urge to get up was mastered by an unwillingness to face what the day might bring, her dream or its end, because she knew she could not have worked any harder or done any better. No, if she didn't get the score needed for Medicine she wouldn't try again. She would be bitterly disappointed, not just for herself, but for the family who had loved and supported her so magnificently, especially over the last twelve months. They deserved her dream every bit as much as she did.

It had been such a strange year, mingling with other people of her own age, or who might have been her age. Her family had settled December the thirteenth as her birthday, the day she came out of the storm, in three days' time. Until that very moment she hadn't given it a thought.

She had initially been afraid that her fellow students, learning she had no past, would think of her as some sort of freak and treat her accordingly.

STORM DANCING

To her surprise they didn't care at all about her past. Indeed, they didn't care about anybody's past. They weren't interested in the past at all. They studied history for the purpose of gaining marks, never thinking to learn from it, or put themselves in its stream. For the same reason they weren't interested in the future either, which really surprised her. Tomorrow hadn't happened, and so why be concerned with it? What mattered was today, what mattered was the moment. Life to them was defined by a succession of individual experiences, some good, some bad, some sweet, some bitter, each one seemingly unconnected to any overall purpose for existence. Storm's worldview was completely different, and it was this which made her strange, and not her lack of memory. Her fellow students soon discovered her unwillingness to embrace such a universal paradigm of life, and concluded she was a fish swimming in a different fish tank altogether.

She was so hot, how much sex did she get every week? None. Boyfriends? Same answer. Girlfriends? Not the way you mean. Never been drunk, never been stoned, never, never, never. In fact the only life experiences she seemed to share with the girls appeared to be eating, breathing and going to class. Her distinctiveness didn't keep them away, however. Had she been able to read their minds, she would have discovered they were drawn to a certain freshness, a joy, an intact clarity of purpose in her, which if they were honest, they knew they didn't possess. The experiences she lacked were the ones which had only added more noise to the cacophony which was their life. Their culture told them the journey was important, not the destination, yet somehow this girl seemed to enjoy the living of one in the light of the other. There was a laughter in her voice, an honesty in her eyes, which lacked the cynicism which had slowly greyed over their own perception of nearly everything. A cynicism which made itself apparent in their practical atheism and their jaundiced view of anything making the ridiculous claim to be truth.

Once she had thought her lack of memory a disadvantage, now she regarded it as an absolute blessing. Perhaps she had been like that too. How incredibly helpful it was to be a follower of the Way and to know who you were and where you were going, even though you didn't even know your real name.

The young men on the other hand, who received a 'no' to every proposition, simply concluded she was secretly gay, and went searching for other hot girls who weren't.

There was no argument about her academic ability however, and being different didn't stop them from coming to her for help at an increasingly annoying rate. Still, it was an opportunity to show them that being a follower of the Way made a difference.

She turned over on her other side, lifted her head and glanced at the alarm clock on her bedside table. Ten o'clock. The mail would have come an hour ago. Best get up and face the music. Come on, Storm, courage.

The door opened and Ellen burst in carrying a cup of tea. "Time to get up," she said brightly. "Too much sleep is really bad for you. Made you some tea."

She plonked the mug down on the bedside table, and whipped the sheet off the bed before Storm had time to grab hold of her only covering, leaving her lying there stark naked. She bounded out of bed and wrapped herself in her dressing gown which lay draped over the back of a chair.

"Ellen!" She scolded. "How many times have I told you not to do that. Imagine what would have happened if Peter had walked in after you."

"Would have made his day," Ellen laughed.

"Well it wouldn't have made mine," Storm retorted crossly.

She tied the cord around her waist and stood studying her sister's beaming face. Ellen was radiating repressed excitement, ready to explode at any second. "What's going on?" she asked.

"Nothing," Ellen said innocently. "Do you want your tea?"

"I'll take it out with me. Anyone in the breakfast room?"

"All gone. Mum and Dad are out and Peter's studying."

"Thanks for waking me up. Second thoughts, I'd better get dressed so I can get the mail."

"I brought it in."

"Was there a letter for me?"

"Forgot to notice."

"For goodness sake, Ellen!" Storm said, even more annoyed. "Don't you know what comes in the mail today?"

Storm grabbed her crutches, wrenched open the door and went a dozen paces down the hall.

She froze, staring.

The entire breakfast room was covered with streamers. There was a cake on the table and a bottle of champagne. Far from being empty, the entire family was there, standing around the table simmering in anticipation.

Seeing her in the doorway, Basa leapt forward with a shriek of excitement and threw her arms around Storm who was quite bewildered. "My darling," she cried, "you did it. You did it."

There were tears in her eyes.

"W...w...what?" Storm stammered, still trying to work out what was going on.

Andrew and Peter ran over and hugged her in turn.

"You've taken eighth place in the whole state, Storm. Your score will get you into anything. I am so, so *proud* of you!" Andrew kissed her head and gave her a huge daddy hug.

"What? I couldn't have... how do you...?" Storm stammered, still trying to grasp the truth.

Ellen raced over to the table and snatched a piece of paper from it. "It's in your letter. I waited an age for the post, and when it came I tore it open. You were stressing out about it, but I knew you'd be brilliant."

Storm stared at the numbers next to her name in a state of shock. She could feel tears streaming down her face. Wiping them away she read the letter again. "Where does it say I came eighth? I can't see…"

"It doesn't say there," Peter laughed, hugging her again and kissing her on the cheek. "The Board of Studies rang half an hour ago and told us. They wanted to speak to you, but as usual Ellen took the call and pretended."

"You didn't," Storm gasped.

"Of course I did, you were asleep," Ellen retorted.

Storm dropped to her knees and hugged her sister. "You're so naughty. I love you."

A champagne cork ricocheted off the ceiling.

"A toast, a toast to an incredibly brave and brilliant young woman." Andrew shouted, handing around the glasses.

"To an incredibly brilliant and beautiful young woman," Peter echoed quietly.

"How did you get the cake? When did all this happen?" Storm waved her arms towards the bunting.

"It was action stations," Ellen explained. "As soon as I got the gen on your score, Dad shot down to the Village. We were hoping you'd stay asleep while we did it. I told Mum to go in and give you a shot of sedative, but she wouldn't. Then you kept on sleeping, and we were all bursting with excitement waiting for you to wake up, so Mum sent me in to give you the treatment."

STORM DANCING

Storm went from one to the other, hugging them ferociously and crying "Thank you, thank you!" Over and over again. "I couldn't have done it without you, done anything without you. I can't tell you how much I love you. I'm so blessed, so incredibly blessed."

The euphoria lasted most of the morning. The head of school at Sydney Institute rang to congratulate Storm for taking out first place, and said they were arranging a special function in her honour early next year. The glass of champagne before breakfast had gone straight to her head, and she hoped she had thanked them coherently on the phone. Uncle Brian rang to say congratulations because they had published the top ten in the paper. Matthew from the Village rang and sounded ecstatic as he congratulated her. He would put the paper up in his supermarket, he said, telling everyone about their resident artist's success. The press rang to organise an interview with all the other top students. Would she mind if someone came round and took her picture? Yes she would. No pictures, please.

Ellen, who had consumed two glasses of champagne before anyone noticed, had taken up residence on the lounge in front of the television, looking incredibly sleepy and making small giggling noises. Andrew and Basa, who had somehow contrived to be at home all day, were busy organising further celebrations.

Peter was finding new ways to say how completely overcome he was with her wonderful success, and unwittingly telling her he loved her every time, which Storm valued even more than his praise. One day she would let him know she adored him, but not yet. Some things had to happen first, and she was rather fearful they never would.

Suddenly Ellen flew through the lounge room door shouting. "Storm! You gotta see this. Come on everyone, quick, quick."

Storm grabbed her crutches and shot into the room followed by Peter and Basa with Andrew not far behind. She turned around to face the television and gasped. It was the Midday Show hosted by none other than Joel Streetman from Good Morning Sydney. Storm had only seen him once, and publicly expressed the view that his infantile attempts at gutter humour made her feel physically nauseous. On the screen were two leather lounge chairs separated by a low table. Joel occupied the right hand one, and in the left sat a carbon copy of Storm herself. She was wearing a light blue designer evening dress, cut high across the back and low across the front, covering her shoulders but not her arms, and allowing the audience ample opportunity to appreciate her shapely legs crossed over in front of her.

Storm stared at the screen in disbelief. "Who is that woman?" she gasped.

"It's Rachel Demarra the actress, you know, the voice of Princess Kalia Jan. She's done some other movies we've never watched, and now she's in Australia for the release of her latest, Portrait of Emily Jones, or something." Ellen obligingly supplied the information she had gleaned before they came into the room.

"How come she looks like me?" Storm demanded loudly.

"Doppelganger. Turn the sound up a bit," Peter said, quite as gob-smacked as Storm was.

Streetman's voice surged into the room. "Now Rachel, some of the viewers mightn't realise you're an Australian yourself with a long acting career in this country. Can you tell us a little about it?"

"I did a lot of stage plays for Harry Donahue," Demarra answered. "He eventually took to the bottle, and it killed him. It was a dreadful time. A budding artist has to take what they can. It's not easy to make an acting career in this country."

"I believe his plays called for a lot of naked appearances. How did you feel about that?"

"I'm completely comfortable with my own body, Joel, and I count it a privilege to use it as a means of artistic expression. I can see you appreciate it too by the way you're staring at me."

"Turn her off," Storm demanded. "What was that word you used, Peter?"

"Doppelganger—"

"I want to hear what she has to say. Leave it on." Ellen protectively snatched the remote off the lounge.

"Err, you are a very beautiful woman, Rachel," Streetman said in a flustered voice.

"You're blushing, Joel. I don't mind doing sex scenes in the altogether. Making love is part of life. Don't you take your clothes off to have sex, Joel, or are you shy and try to do it with them on?"

"Ah… that would be… no, I mean, yes. I take them off." Beads of sweat appeared on Streetman's brow. "I believe you spend quite a lot of time in bed with your co-star in Emily Jones."

"Emily is a passionate woman."

Streetman continued. "Some critics have suggested your superb performance as Emily Jones, a passionate woman whose love life comes into conflict with caring for her daughter after she is incapacitated in a train wreck, is due to your own personal experience with—"

"Why Joel," Demarra interrupted. "You know that subject is off limits, it says so in the contract I signed for this interview. Perhaps you can't read. How would you like me to appear naked on your show? Would that spice up your flagging ratings a bit?"

"Ha, ha," Streetman laughed. "Our viewers might think – hey, what are you doing?"

Ms. Demarra had stood up from her chair, taken off her microphone, and was in the act of slowly and seductively unzipping her dress down the back. Streetman sprang up with the face of a man who knows his next job will be sweeping streets. He began to flap his arms around in a pathetic attempt to dissuade his eager guest from revealing all.

Undeterred, the dress fell to the floor.

Underneath Ms. Demarra was wearing a rather small red and white designer bikini. There was no doubt at all about her superb figure, and Peter, watching with his mouth half open, remembered where he had seen a perfect replica of that figure before. She slinked seductively towards Streetman, pushed him back into his chair, sat down on his lap, and draped one arm languorously around his shoulder. The studio audience hooted their approval loudly.

Streetman made a last desperate effort to regain control of his own show. "I must say you gave us all a scare then, Rachel."

"Gave you a scare, did I, Joel darling?" Demarra purred. "Must be the after effects of that naughty little joint you smoked before you went on camera this morning. You need another mint. Do we have one in here?"

"W... what? I didn't..." Streetman blustered.

Rachel slipped her hand inside his coat, and retrieved a little metal tin of mints. She opened it and pushed one in between his lips with a long finger. "That's better." She stroked his chin with her outstretched hand. "Isn't this what you wanted? Of course you did. Your heart's racing in anticipation."

She plucked the microphone off Streetman's lapel, and slipped it under his shirt against his chest. A quick thumping sound came through the speaker.

The audience went wild.

She pulled the microphone out and clipped it onto his shirt, all with the same languorous movement, and began to stroke his hair. "What would you like to do if all these cameras weren't flashing, and this wonderful audience had all gone home?" she asked in a soft, sexy voice. "How about it, Joel, shall we tell the viewers how you react when a beautiful woman in a bikini sits on your lap? Working up a little sweat are we?"

Storm lunged across the room and yanked the power cord out of its socket.

"Turn it back on! I want to see what she does to him next," Ellen shouted, bounding off the lounge.

"I'd rather die," Storm shuddered. "How embarrassing. She looks just like me all the way down. Yuk. No. What a dreadful thought. How revolting. It couldn't be, could it? Please say no."

"She's a doppelganger, Storm," Peter said consolingly, "someone unrelated who looks like you, that's all."

"There couldn't be... you know... could there? She's been living in America, hasn't she? It isn't possible is it?" Storm's face wore the horror expressed in her voice.

"Of course not," Andrew chimed in from the doorway. "You might look like the woman, but that's where it ends. Think, Storm, you're totally different in every other way."

"She's without shame!" Storm said vehemently. "I never thought I'd ever feel sorry for Streetman, but I just did. She made a complete fool of him. He didn't know which way was up in the end."

"She out-sleazed him for once and good on her," Ellen said with a giggle. "I think she's pretty smart as well as being comfortable with her own body. I feel comfortable with mine."

Ellen adopted a provocative pose. She turned her head on one side, attempting a seductive expression, then spoilt it all by dissolving into giggles and falling back on the lounge.

Basa was frowning. "Comfortable with her own body? What's that supposed to mean? Being brazen enough to flaunt it naked before the world? Storm's right, the woman's without shame. Art, my eye. We know why that sort of thing draws an audience, and it's got nothing to do with art."

"Thanks, Mum," Storm said with a shiver. "Ugh. Fancy being related to her. I've gone all cold inside. You really don't suppose..."

285

"Of course not, darling," Basa soothed. "Peter's right, she's your doppelganger, that's all. Everybody has one somewhere in the world. In med school there was a girl who looked exactly like me. I was always afraid Andrew would notice."

"Sally Mackenzie," Andrew chuckled. "She might have had your face, but not your mind or your heart, my darling."

"No?"

"You know I only ever saw one woman in med school."

Basa turned her face up towards Andrew who folded her into his arms and covered her lips in a long passionate kiss.

"Now that's more like it," Ellen giggled.

CHAPTER 30

Westmead Research Centre, three years before the Storm

Isaac Gilead surveyed the conference room of shocked faces.

"A human head?" Yanac exploded. What in God's Name do you mean?"

Lavro Festerhaus broke into laughter. "He's bought a frozen head. Cut off and dropped into ice. Why didn't you ask? I could have brought you one of those really cheap. Happens all the time where I come from."

"Nothing so useless, my dear Lavro," Gilead replied, still smiling. "What use would frozen tissue be to us? These experiments must in the end involve *in vivo* transplants, not *in vitro* ones."

Kevin Lucknow gripped his neck in both hands and made a severing movement, laughing out loud. "He's got his severed head attached to some heart – lung machine. It's probably circulating the blood of the deceased. Reminds me of C.S. Lewis – That Hideous Strength. I must congratulate you, Professor. No doubt our nursing colleagues will enjoy turning on its oxygen so it can speak to us, and brushing its teeth every night."

The aforementioned nurses, all ten of them, wished they had taken Gilead's offer of exit. Everyone else was laughing out loud including the man himself. An unbalanced ghoul, and they were locked into working with him. What a terrible fate. A stir of voices began to grow.

"A severed head, fed with its own blood by some machine? Nothing as outlandish, Kevin," Gilead said, smiling. "No, we have been the beneficiaries of an extraordinary gift, a functioning cortical tissue library with its own support system, ready for *in vivo* experimentation. At present it has sustained some damage, which is all to the good, because we will concentrate on those areas first. It is this unique acquisition which persuaded ARG to finance the project at enormous cost to themselves."

"Which they will recap a thousandfold over if we succeed," Lucknow chuckled.

"They'll make billions. No wonder they don't mind investing a million or two." Ross echoed Lucknow's comment.

Hargraves cut in. "What exactly do you mean by a tissue library? Frozen embryo? What support system, human, animal? Has the company sanctioned this?"

"Why don't you come and see?" Gilead was bursting with excitement. "Oh, before you leave this room, please make sure the paperwork in front of each one of you is signed – a short legal document forbidding you to discuss anything you learn or see within this research centre with anyone else. ARG insisted on it, I'm afraid, and I do suggest you take their threat of legal action seriously."

There was a general rustling of paper along with a soft muttering, which could have been low voiced complaint, but nobody showed any hesitation to sign. Their professional curiosity was bursting at the seams. In a very short time a team of thirty five pairs of feet followed Gilead out of the room, down the corridor, through the imaging lab. They stopped at the air lock into the sterile room beyond.

"Each time you enter this sterile facility you must gown up," Gilead instructed. "That includes all support staff and technicians."

He took a package enclosed in a plastic envelope off a nearby chair to demonstrate. "In the air lock there is a large rack of these and a chute for disposal. You open them – so – by pulling this tab. There are also covers for your shoes and breathing masks. The lock can only accommodate five people at a time, so it will take a while to get us all through. When the first group has gowned and gloved, please press the exit button into the sterile area. Only then will the entrance be enabled. The air lock is flushed with sterile air and disinfectant mist. I hope none of you are asthmatic. Please wait for the rest before you explore."

Half an hour passed before all those in the conference room stood gowned, capped and gloved inside the sterile room. One end was equipped with a modern operating theatre. At the other end an area was screened off with a removable curtain. Gilead advanced towards this and threw it aside. In the space beyond was a single hospital bed, and on the bed, visible above the sheet, was a shaved head. There was an audible gasp from thirty two throats. Gilead advanced on the bed and removed the sheet, revealing the naked body of a rather podgy teenage girl. A urinary catheter tube protruded from between her legs, a central line above her left breast, and a cannula needle from an artery in her left leg.

A shaken Ross was the first to speak. "My God, Gilead. The girl's breathing. She's alive! You don't mean we are going to experiment on her brain? What bioethics committee sanctioned this?"

"My esteemed colleague," Gilead replied in a very level voice, "this is no longer a young woman, and it will be most unhelpful if you regard it as such. The young woman she was is dead. I have a copy of her death certificate. She has also been officially cremated. What remains is tissue library twenty nine, so named because it became available on the twenty ninth of a certain month, which I will not divulge. It comes here by the ingenuity of Doctor Ferris, to whom we are impossibly indebted."

He walked over to the bedside and touched the girl's cranium.

"In here is our tissue library, ready for experimentation. This" – he waved his hand over the girl's torso - "is our library's support system. In order for our tissue library to be maintained in useful condition, this support system must be kept in excellent functioning order. This is why there are two expert nutritionists, and three expert physiotherapists on our team. The library is operating on the barest level of consciousness necessary to maintain homeostasis, temperature, blood flow, and respiration. Our two expert physiotherapists will need to use electrostimulation as well as massage to maintain muscle tone and prevent wastage."

He touched the girl's bare head once again.

"When we have decided on our approach we will open our library, extract some of the damaged frontal cortex, and begin the process of neuron replacement. We will close it up again, and monitor progress using the advanced technology next door. When sufficient time has elapsed, we will open our library again and sample the new tissue, record changes, and determine our success or failure. The imaging lab will be able to tell us if the transplanted neurons have connected into existing cortical circuitry. If the support system does not fail, we should be able to do this until we have learned how to regrow every single structure."

Gilead beamed at his astonished audience. "If we succeed, colleagues, those diseases I mentioned in my introduction will begin to vanish into memory. This is our challenge. We shall never have another opportunity like this. It is imperative the support system does not deteriorate in any manner whatsoever. It must be kept totally healthy. Its immune systems must be maintained, least it succumb to some virus which has managed to get past our sterile protocols. If we lose our library, this project will terminate, and our efforts be totally for naught. I trust those members of our support staff understand the critical nature of their role."

He paused, fixed Ross with a steady eye. "Oh, and for your information, David, the Australian Bioethics Committee has never heard of this project."

"You're taking one hell of a risk," Ross muttered, obviously distressed.

"What level of incapacity did this – this tissue library possess when you wheeled her – it – in here? I trust she – it – wasn't capable of returning to consciousness?"

"Would it have mattered?" Metzger turned sharply towards the speaker. "Your attitude concerns me, Ross. The girl you seem so worried about is dead. Her parents have grieved, are moving on with their lives. We are dealing with a discarded piece of broken human machinery which no longer even possesses a name. One which we can learn from. There are over three hundred thousand Australians suffering from dementia right now, and this is expected to increase to almost half a million by the end of the decade. Where lie your scruples? As Isaac said, this is a tissue library, maintained by a support system, nothing more. A tissue library which could possibly bring relief to millions of suffering human beings. Be thankful you have been given the extraordinary privilege of taking part in this research."

Metzger shook his head and turned away from Ross whose face was slowly colouring, whether with embarrassment or rage it was hard to tell.

Gilead lifted his gaze from the figure on the bed and spoke. His voice was quiet, and unlike Metzger there was no trace of anger in his face or his reply. "Doctor Ross, the project was never put before the Australian Bioethics Committee, for the simple reason it would have been rejected. Not on any rational grounds, but on some nonsense couched in terms of human dignity, respect for human life, interfering with the soul, and so on. There is no soul, learned colleagues. The human mind is a machine, a wonderful, complex machine, the like of which there is no parallel on Earth, but a machine, nothing more. Let us take this opportunity and learn how to repair it. As for dignity, you are all familiar with the pathology of CNS diseases. Do any of these enhance human dignity? No. In every case human dignity is diminished all the way down to zero. Even if our tissue library had walked in here fully conscious and functioning - which it did not - it seems to me that one life lost for the sake of millions of others is hardly unethical. The odds in war are far less persuasive, yet we glory in those. Should we not rejoice in this, the opportunity to take a ruined machine, and use it to restore the dignity of so many others?"

To this reply no one gave answer. A few heads nodded, others simply stared at Gilead, their thoughts impossible to read. Ross shrugged his shoulders, his face still a bright shade of pink. A few of the nurses and two of the physiotherapists seemed unhappy.

Lucknow was grinning ear to ear. "I guess John and I are going to be pretty busy with our nice toys. I should be able to resolve cranial function down to less than a square millimetre, that's if John keeps his bloody fluorine-eighteen or oxygen-fifteen away from my balls."

"Why thank you Kevin. If you find your tea strangely warm one day you'll know why." John Roberts was taciturn at the best of times, and very allergic to radioactive isotope jokes.

Gilead cleared his throat gently for silence. "As you can see, our tissue library's support system is already in need of constant care. I would ask the nurses and other medical support staff if they would meet me in the conference room in, let's say, half an hour, where we will discuss your duties in detail. I would like exhaustive tests run on the toys, as you put it, Kevin. John, if you would calibrate the detectors for fluorine-eighteen. I think we will monitor dopamine receptors first, just to determine the amount of damage in our library and where it is. Doctor Yung, would you be good enough to go with them, please?"

He motioned the group towards the air lock. "Every morning there will be a compulsory briefing in the conference room at eight a.m. for those not rostered on duty. These meetings will be used to report progress and determine further work. That will be all for now, thank you."

The team began to head towards the air lock. Two men remained. Metzger turned to his old friend with a sigh. "Even the finest intellectual minds cannot agree on the simplest ethical questions. I wonder if there is any hope for the human race. What think you, Isaac?"

"Yes, I was aware of the tension," Isaac said softly, "and I will speak to those involved, though I don't really believe I will change their minds. So irrational, so unhelpful this clinging to some non-existent metaphysical reality. I think I will find Ross is a believer in the human soul, although of course, he will give me no rational reason for it. Two of our physiotherapists might even be secretly religious, although we tried to purge that deadly trait at interview. I hope the team will be able to embrace our goals and function as a whole without allowing such nonsense to interfere."

He gazed at the tissue library on the bed, and spoke to it, never expecting a reply. "You have been chosen for greatness, young one. You may have finished your own journey on earth, but the one you are now embarked upon will be remembered for generations to come."

"Talking to our tissue library now are we? You'd better not let any of the others catch you philosophising by the bedside," Metzger chuckled quietly. He took Gilead by the arm. "Come, my friend, I feel like a good coffee, and I may be able to find a small something to add to it."

CHAPTER 31

The initial briefing occurred the next day at precisely eight a.m. Two nursing staff, one of the dieticians and Max Hargraves, had been rostered on patient care that morning. The rest were all there, sitting up with their notebooks, pens poised in their hands.

"Colleagues," Gilead began, "I am aware that not all of you – I refer to our excellent nurses and technicians – are familiar with the advanced biochemistry and genetics we are going to employ in the initial pursuit of our goal. I will try to make matters as simple as possible. After this meeting, I would ask the academic portion of our team to remain so we can add further detail. In short, this is how we intend to proceed."

Gilead turned to the board and wrote 'A.S.C.' in large blue letters.

"Our starting place is the acquisition of appropriate stem cells," he continued. "We could have used embryonic omnipotent cells, harvested from aborted foetuses, but there are genetic complications to these as well as availability problems. No, we are going to obtain our initial stem cells by autologous[2] harvesting our support system's adipose tissue, something it has in abundant supply."

---

[2] tissue taken from the same individual

"But those are multipotent adult stem cells, not neural stem cells at all." Ross raised the first objection.

"Doctor Ross is perfectly correct," Gilead replied, "but neural stem cells are also adult stem cells. We will take these harvested cells and genetically modify them to produce neurospheres of neuroepithelial cells, and allow these to multiply without differentiation."

"By what process?" This time Lavro Festerhaus was quick with the question.

"Our esteemed colleague Professor Metzger has pioneered a method which I am sure will succeed—"

Metzger interrupted. "What Isaac should have said, is Professor Gilead has pioneered a method which has already been shown to work, in which I have played a small advisory role."

"You are far too self-effacing, Gerhardt my friend," Gilead smiled warmly towards his colleague. "Sufficient to say we have almost perfected this part of the process. Kevin and John have already identified the areas of damage in our tissue library, and we will begin with these. In fact more than a third of the frontal lobe on both hemispheres is severely damaged. When we have cultured sufficient neural stem cells for our purpose, we will treat those parts of the prefrontal cortex with a virus. This will cause the healthy neurons and associated glial cells to emit the correct environmental marker signals. This done, we will inject our cultured cells into the damaged cortex, where we hope they will now differentiate into neurons and associated cells, repairing the damage. Hopefully, these new neurons will connect into the existing cortical circuitry. That in a nutshell is the process. In fact it is a little more complicated. Our first task is the harvesting, then us geneticists will be busy for a time. Are there any questions?"

There weren't.

"Good," Gilead said, replacing his whiteboard marker in the tray. "The autologous harvesting will take place in half an hour. The support system is being prepped as we speak."

The operation went smoothly. A large volume of lipids were extracted by liposuction. The geneticists took them into the biochemistry labs to begin the process of separating out the stem cells, all talking excitedly together and using very long words while they did it. Hargraves checked the support system's post-surgical state, and laid down careful instructions for the nursing staff and the two dieticians. Recovery should be swift, but they were to keep an eye out for the slightest hint of infection or complications.

Three days later the physiotherapists were let loose on its limbs, massaging, electrostimulating, ensuring there was no muscle wastage.

Pat Cornish, who was working on the support system's thigh muscle at the time, turned to Sally Brown who was massaging its left leg, a couple of electrodes attached across the muscle. "Never massaged a support system before," she muttered. "Feels just like a girl's leg to me."

"Don't let them hear you say that. Just hang in here for five years and buy a dream with your pay," Sally whispered.

"Can't help it," Pat scowled. "Poor little thing. I bet her tummy feels really sore right now. See all that bruising, and there's swelling too. I think I'm hurting her by lifting her leg like this."

"She can't feel it," Sally said quickly. "Just as well. You must admit she looks a bit better for the loss of all that podge."

"Who says she can't feel it?" Pat retorted angrily. "My mother was in a coma for weeks before she died. I always thought she could hear me, even though she couldn't say so. I really hope this poor little girl can't hear what they're saying in her presence. I'd be absolutely terrified. And what will happen if their tissue implants go wrong? What will she become then? Some sort of monster."

"I suspect they'll never let her return to consciousness to find out." Sally grimaced at the thought.

"What do you mean by that?" Pat snapped.

"When you've finished with a lab rat what do you do with it?" Another grimace.

"They wouldn't!" Pat's horrified eyes bored into her colleague.

"Want to bet your salary on that?"

"I wish I'd said no," Pat confided. "Tony and I have only been married a year, and we thought this would be a great way to get our own home and start a family so I could be a full time mum. This was a dreadful mistake."

"As I said, just keep doing what we're told, and in five years or less we'll be out of here." Sally gave Pat's arm a meaningful squeeze.

"Less?"

"Perhaps their experiments will destroy the support system. If that brain stops completely her heart will stop too."

"I hope it does, poor little girl," Pat said bitterly.

Further conversation was cut short by the approach of Doctor Hargraves. "How is the muscle tissue?" he asked.

"Seeing she can't tell me, I'd say it could do with a lot more electrostimulation," Pat Cornish answered sharply. "Sally and I are working on it."

"Support system, not she," Hargraves cautioned. "Be careful you don't get confused. I need a more detailed report. In twenty minutes, with strategies, in my office."

The two women eyed one another. There was no doubt about the way the land would lie for the duration of their sentence. They were right at the bottom of the pecking order, and they had better get used to it.

It took four months before the neural stem cells had progressed to the point where the geneticists were happy to begin the process of transplantation. The transplant began on a Monday at eight twenty a.m. Gilead was chief surgeon with Ross assisting. Hargraves was the anaesthetist, whose job it was to make certain there were no spurious impulses sent back into the support system when the library was incised. Four of the nurses were selected for theatre duty, four more to implement recovery procedures. The remaining geneticists were standing by in the biochemistry lab. Kevin Lucknow had been told to make sure his toys were ready at a moment's notice to perform a standard MRI, and the physiotherapists could take the day off.

The first incision took place at eight thirty seven. An hour later, with the skull opened, Gilead cut a portion of the damaged cortex out of both lobes, and Ross applied the virus to the surrounding tissue. Now they had to wait until the correct markers were released by the affected neurons. Ross kept taking samples for the geneticists to analyse. When they were satisfied, Gilead took the prepared sample of neural stem cells and injected them into their prepared places. The skull bones were replaced, the scalp tissue folded back and stitched very carefully by Ross. Before he specialised in genetics, he had been a superb plastic surgeon. Gilead had chosen his team with care.

The library was bandaged carefully and wheeled into recovery. The four nurses kept a careful watch on it, recording practically everything including constant brain activity. The surgery required to open the head meant quite a lot of blood escaped into facial tissue, causing severe bruising. Those, and the large bandages around the cranium, turned the support system into a rather sad spectacle. The sight would have wrung pity out of any caring heart. Care but not pity was required, they were told.

The four recovery nurses, staring at the poor, bruised little face, felt pity by the spadeful.

The eight a.m. conference on Tuesday morning received a report from Kevin to say there was no dangerous cranial bleeding. The recovery nursing team confirmed the support system was stable. The geneticists told the meeting they were quietly optimistic the transgenic neural stem cells would differentiate properly.

A week later, the physiotherapists were brought back to do the job they increasingly hated. For the next two months optimism amongst the geneticists began to grow. The support system's vital signs remained within limits, and Lucknow reported the new cells were growing into new cortical tissue.

❋ ❋ ❋

The very next day Sarah Gleeson, one of the day care nurses, recorded unusual fluctuations in support system temperature, which she could neither account for nor control. Antibiotics were prescribed and administered. Still the temperature continued to fluctuate in an unpredictable and sometimes alarming manner. The following day an irregular heart rate added to their concerns. Gilead was informed immediately and scheduled John Roberts to perform PET tests, assuming the fluctuations were caused by the new cortical cells connecting to existing neural circuitry in some fashion.

The following morning, at the regular meeting they learned the truth.

"John and I have performed extensive tests," Lucknow said evenly, "and we are happy to report the new transplanted cells have differentiated into cortex. In fact they've differentiated so well they're taking over the existing cortical structures."

A round of applause from all.

"Yes," Roberts continued, "and the new cortex is beginning to connect to existing neural circuits. I can trace the activity easily."

"Well, I guess congratulations are due," Ross said.

"They certainly are," Lucknow grinned. "You've made the first human rabbit in history. Doctor Moreau would be proud."

"What the hell do you mean?" Metzger jumped to his feet, his face black with rage. "How dare you pour your ill-witted cynicism over eminent scientists far more accomplished than yourself."

If Lucknow was perturbed by Metzger's rage, he totally failed to show it. The smile still lingered on his face. In fact it strengthened into a definite chuckle. "Dear Gerhardt, the cynicism is all on the side of the eminent geneticists like yourself. The witches brew you stuffed into your tissue library has resolved into a large three-layered olfactory cortex. It's making a growing number of quite bizarre connections with the white matter below, and your support system is probably trying to smell with its tits. Given a few more months, you might even begin to notice its nose twitching. The nutritionists should change the diet to carrot juice."

A gasp of horror echoed throughout the room. Lucknow was still chuckling to himself. The others present didn't seem to appreciate the funny side of the situation at all. The nurses looked pale and shocked. The three physiotherapists simply stared aghast.

Gilead was on his feet, his voice trembling with rage. "Show me the negatives. How dare you bring these findings to this meeting! Why was I not informed the instant you had run the tests?"

"Because you only ordered the tests yesterday and we ran them late last night. You and Metzger were out on the town, remember, celebrating your impending rabbit morphing success." Lucknow was still laughing to himself.

Gilead glared at Lucknow as though he would have liked to have his cortex fried and served with toast for breakfast. "We must determine what is to be done," he said, trying valiantly to control his anger. "Any of our support staff who wish to leave are free to do so at this point."

Nobody moved a muscle.

"Very well," Gilead continued. "The NSC's are differentiating incorrectly, but they are still making cortical tissue. This is an enormous advance in its own right."

"With horrific consequences," Ross interrupted. "You led me to believe the differentiation would be perfect. Instead we've created a gross abnormality in a human brain. Surely we should have used a mouse or rhesus model first."

"Bit late for that, isn't it?" Lucknow laughed. "Want to know what I think? The NSC's were bodgie to start with. The three witches cooked up their brew by the light of the wrong moon. Perhaps they added too much eye of newt, or more probably they began with the wrong sort of stem cells in the first place."

"Leaving aside your crass attempts at humour, Lucknow, just what sort of stem cells would you have started with?" Gilead was dangerously close to losing his temper.

"Embryonic neural stem cells of course."

"Where do you suppose we could obtain those with compatible genetic information?" Gilead protested.

"Simple," Lucknow said. "Inject your support system with fertility hormone and get it pregnant. Wait a month or two and harvest away. You could repeat the process every few months until you're swimming in embryos. I'd even volunteer my services – and waive the stud fee."

"You're revolting!" Sarah Gleeson shouted, her face black with rage.

"Doctor Lucknow's suggestion is not without merit," Metzger said evenly, "even though some of you find it offensive. But the problem is not the neural stem cells – which differentiated into cortical tissue. The problem, may I remind you, is they differentiated into the wrong sort of tissue. I take your point, Ross, and I disagree with it. Some of the finest minds in genetics and neurology are in this room. We have a problem to solve. Please restrict your comments to this task. If you can't do that, leave now."

There was total silence. The horrified expression on the faces of the physiotherapists, and most of the nursing staff remained. Some of them stood up to leave, because they knew they could contribute nothing to the discussion and didn't want to hear it anyway.

Surprisingly it was Ross who made the first useful suggestion. "Did anyone monitor homeodomain transcription factors, particularly Lhx2? If this transcription factor was absent before our neuroepithelial cells made the transition into radial glia, I would expect the differentiation to produce an anomalous result."

Gilead stared at Ross for a long time. "My friend, we may not agree as to the model, but your suggestion is quite brilliant. Neither have we checked the levels of fibroblast growth factor, such as Fgf10 protein which regulates this entire process. Most remiss. Gentlemen, I believe Doctor Ross has identified the problem. Let's run with his suggestion, and modify our implant technique. We will have to remove the invasive tissue as soon as possible. Shall we adjourn to the biochemistry lab?"

The meeting in the biochemistry lab lasted until two a.m. the following morning.

❀ ❀ ❀

Three days later the tissue library was re-opened. The spurious cortex formation was removed and replaced with a new culture of neuroepithelial cells. Once again the recovery nurses monitored the support system intensively for three weeks, but this time there were no apparent problems. Two months later, Gilead was able to announce to the team at the usual eight a.m. meeting, that as far as they could tell without removing some of the new cortical tissue, the transplant had been completely successful. The cells had differentiated properly, and the new pre-frontal tissue was apparently connecting itself into the existing circuitry.

A week later the library was opened again and samples of the new cortex removed for rigorous testing which confirmed their optimism.

Gilead and his team had, for the first time in medical history, managed to replace damaged prefrontal cortex.

The conference that morning was turned into a time of celebration. Even the physiotherapists shared the overall excitement. The results were sent back to ARG so that they could join in the celebration as well, which they did, apparently, because every member of staff received a substantial bonus in their next pay.

Over the next eighteen months the team managed to replace all the library's prefrontal cortex, damaged and undamaged, with the transplanted material. The only difference seemed to be that the new cortex was far more convoluted than the old, and the neural density was over eight percent greater. What that meant in actual terms, nobody was prepared to say.

Then the serious trouble began.

CHAPTER 32

Gilead's office, like all the others in the complex, was totally without windows, its only lighting provided by architecturally designed halogen fixtures mounted high on the walls, which threw patches of whiteness on the smooth ceiling. To this had been added a large desk lamp, its stark blue-white fluorescence casting sharp shadows in contrast to the diffuse mellow warmth from above. The desk was littered deep with journals and reports, the whiteboard at the end of the room covered with complex biochemistry. On the other wall the latest negatives from the MRI and PET machines hung in front of translucent white panels, now switched off. On the opposite wall Gilead had hung a large picture of the Jordan River, where the narrow stream had widened out into a large pool lined with reedy grasses. He was staring at it now, contemplating the long and often turbulent journey which had led him from his home until now. So much struggle, so much pain, yet he had succeeded, and his success would one day go down into the annals of medical history.

> 'Gilead and his team were the first to demonstrate that all cortical structures could be replaced by genetically modified adult stem cells, and so began one of the greatest advances in modern medicine, the successful treatment of neural disease...'

He remembered the terrible visits to his own father, a brilliant man who could not even remember his son's name. Six long years of suffering, seeing the man he loved slowly but surely diminish into a pathetic figure who had to be fed and taken to the toilet, wheeled around, dressed, a witless shadow of the fine mind and joyful character he once possessed. His death had been a blessing, his mother tired and worn out with sorrow. Yet that experience had determined his son's life direction. He would find a cure, and he had. The tissue library had been totally repaired, totally. For the first time he was struck with the significance of his silent words.

Repaired, yes, it had been. A totally new frontal cortex, one without any prior programming of any sort, without any environmental conditioning. A brain without any culturally injected irrationality. A mind free from the pernicious prejudice of religion, a spirit who could once again join the human race and contribute to its greatness. Yes, a living mind which he had built, his greatest single advocate and testimony. For an insane second he thought to bring her back to consciousness, just so he could watch her face when he told her. "I built your mind, child. I built it so you could live and be what you were meant to be, to fulfil your true purpose. I set you free from the curse of irrationality, of superstition, of fear, of subservience to some non-existent god."

He imagined the love and adoration in her eyes. He heard her voice begging him, "teach me, maker of my mind, teach me to think like you. Teach me to be what you have made me to be." He shook his head free from the vision. There was more to be done, much more. He had yet to learn how to replace other cortical structures. Now was not the time to lose focus, and yet... and yet...

His reverie was interrupted by a knock at the door. Lucknow and Roberts entered on his request. They might not be bosom friends, but they had certainly learned to work together.

"There's something we thought you should know," Lucknow said. "John and I think it's a bit odd, but no doubt an expert neurologist like yourself will find it mundane and boring."

Gilead always found Lucknow intensely irritating, more so because he had interrupted his flight of fantasy. "What?" he asked, annoyed. "Not some more spurious growth?"

"No, nothing like that," Lucknow said evenly. "It's your new-fangled cortex. It's very busy."

"Busy? How do you mean, busy?"

"It's firing off all over the place, accessing neural networks to other structures as well," Lucknow continued. "Of course it reaches a dead end every time it tries to twitch motor neurons because of that lovely cocktail you keep it sucking on every day. Sensory data might be getting through though. You should tell those nurses to use more deodorant."

Gilead winced. Somehow Lucknow, whether intentionally or not had the knack of raising his blood pressure with hardly a word.

Roberts continued. "It's almost as if it's thinking, you know, like you would expect a normal brain to be, and it seems to be doing an awful lot of it."

"Thank you for telling me," Gilead said. "Perhaps the new cortex is formatting itself in some way, you know, like we format a new hard disk. This is a brand new situation, old cortical structures from birth interfacing with the new material. Perhaps this is normal procedure under these circumstances."

"There's something else you ought to know about," Roberts said. "We reported these findings to Ross, and he's been talking to some of the others. He's rather of the opinion you ought to terminate further experimentation and allow the organism to return to consciousness. He feels there's every chance it will."

Gilead frowned deeply. "These others, do they feel that way too?"

Lucknow gave his usual infuriating chuckle. "Metzger is incensed at the suggestion. He's using Gestapo tactics on the believers right now. Ross told him to piss off, but some converts among the nurses have abandoned their love for humanity in favour of retaining their salaries. Festerhaus and Ferris want to keep playing games, and the nutritionists have joined the physiotherapists at the barricades."

"There can be no suggestion we abandon the project," Gilead snapped, banging the table in front of him. "There are more structures in the library which we must learn to replace. When we have completed our work—"

"That's the interesting bit," Lucknow interrupted. "When you've totally replaced its brain what then? Time to give the lab rat a tiny injection and feed it into the incinerator?"

"I find that suggestion highly offensive, Lucknow!" Gilead exploded.

"Merely consistent with your tissue library concept, Herr Professor. When you've read all the books and learnt all there is to know, it's usually time for the shredder. Personally, I'd try to sell off its organs. Makes anonymous disposal easier and turns a profit we could all share in on the side. People pay heaps of shekels for young healthy hearts, lungs, kidneys, eyes, stuff like that. I'm sure ARG wouldn't object to a little entrepreneurial activity."

"There will be none of that," Gilead hissed, on the verge of losing his temper. "If you've finished your report I have work to do."

"Work on, Professor. We bid thee adieu."

Lucknow made a small bow, and the two men went out of the room, leaving Gilead pondering the last suggestion. Dismember his library and support system? What would happen when they had eventually finished with her? He had never given thought to the eventuality. It made perfect logical sense to use her organs for the benefit of others, yet somehow he found the idea repulsive. He imagined himself as the surgeon administering the fatal injection, removing her eyes and heart, eyes which could have opened onto a new world, a heart which could have pulsed to the cause of reason, rejoicing in the new life it had been given. On the other hand, how could a brand new person rise, as it were, like phoenix from the ashes, without bringing discredit on the same brilliant scientists who had brought about her resurrection? A conundrum, but one for some other time, not today. There was work to be done.

There may have been more work to be done, but the conundrum he had so willingly relegated to the future turned up with a vengeance in the eight a.m. conference the following morning.

It began with a politely worded plea from Ross.

"Professor Gilead, you and the other scientists working on this project have already pushed the frontiers of medicine far into the future, repairing a badly damaged prefrontal cortex. This is surely an incredible achievement which will be associated with your name and the names of these other eminent gentlemen for many generations to come."

He paused, spread his hands out towards the others in an imploring gesture. "But this is just my point, we have repaired the cortex. When this young woman came in here she was so badly damaged it was doubtful she could ever have returned from her comatose state. Now there is every possibility of her returning, not only to life, but life unimpaired with any sort of intellectual disability, although this remains to be seen."

He repeated the gesture. "I believe the purpose of medicine is to heal, to make whole, and this is what we have done. I can see no ethical justification for keeping her unconscious when she might well return to an unimpaired and useful life. I believe we should allow her to do just that."

Metzger was quick to reply. "We have had this out before, Ross. This project was set up with the goal of replacing, not just the prefrontal cortex, but every structure in the human brain. We have succeeded with the prefrontal lobes, but the others are untouched. Parkinson's disease has to do with dopamine producing cells dying in the substantia nigra. Stroke can also affect the temporal or occipital lobe. We cannot replace these – yet. More research is needed. Granted we have had a significant success, but the gift of this tissue library is not to be thrown away on one success. No, we must continue our research."

"But she's healthy. She can come back to consciousness. You can't do experiments on a healthy young woman. It's downright immoral!" Sally Brown objected loudly.

"We have done something very wonderful here, and I admit I didn't go along with it in the beginning. But to continue, to remove healthy tissue from her head and experiment on it as though she was... was a... lab rat is ... unethical. Foul!"

"Metzger is right, you haven't any choice." Ferris was on his feet. "Don't forget the girl who sourced this tissue library is dead, dead and cremated. If she suddenly returns to life there will be a lot of eminent scientists in gaol, including me. She has to leave this research facility in the same condition she entered, dead."

"You can't be serious," Bill Lowery exploded, jumping to his feet. "How come a living human being was issued a death certificate in the first place? Seems to me there's people here who should be in gaol already."

"It's here because Ferris body snatched it out of hospital and sensibly wrote a death certificate," Lucknow said. "And I agree, it has to stay dead. When we've all become famous for repairing damaged brains, we sell off its organs and make a little profit on the side. Either that or we keep breeding it, and harvesting its embryonic stem cells for pleasure and profit. Us men could all take turns and widen the genetic pool."

"You amoral piece of shit!" Pat Cornish screamed, standing up so quickly her chair tumbled over behind her. "I've seen the way you ogle her when you feed her naked body into that MRI machine with your wandering hands. Don't tell me you haven't. We're talking about a young woman, not a lab rat or a battery hen. How can you think like this?"

Gilead banged on the table with his coffee cup so hard it shattered into pieces. "There's been enough of this," he shouted. "I understand how some of you may feel, but we persevere. This opportunity does not come every day. We have done great work, but more work needs to be done before we dispose of our library in some painless and appropriate manner. If it helps you, regard her as a wonderful young woman who has given up her possibility of life for the sake of millions of others, and help her make the sacrifice worthwhile."

He stood and glared at the collection of angry faces in front of him.

"Tomorrow we will remove a section of the motor cortex on the edge of the frontal lobe on the left hemisphere. We will inject our prepared stem cells and monitor the results." He held up his hand. "There will be no more discussion. I remind you of the conditions under which you were employed. ARG will not hesitate to adopt punitive measures should anyone feel the urge to sabotage this research. I'm sorry to bring this matter before you. Please, try to see the larger picture."

Half the nurses, all the nutritionists and physiotherapists, together with a large contingent of other support staff stood up and walked out of the room, tight lipped and furious. They had read their contracts thoroughly by now, and knew any breach meant financial ruin, even a lengthy period in gaol.

Safely out of earshot in the corridor, Sally turned to Bill with fire in her eyes. "What do I do every day?" she hissed. "Massage a lab rat? A tissue library? No. I work on the muscles belonging to a young woman, a beautiful young woman, someone who could bloody well walk out of here if it wasn't for these bloody ghouls of butchers who can't see what they're actually contemplating – premeditated murder."

"Yes, but if it wasn't for those ghouls she'd be dead or in some deplorable home for the severely retarded." Bill gave an involuntary shudder. "I think I'd rather never come to consciousness than wake up and be so much less than human." He shook his head. "I find I'm in a bit of a conundrum."

"Besides that, what are we going to do about it?" Pat's face reflected the anger in Sally's. "We tweet a word about what's going on in here and ARG are likely to have us as their next tissue library. I wouldn't put anything past them. Frankly, I'm scared. These people are desperate. Gilead, Metzger and the other academic ghouls in here are desperate to finish the job at any cost. Ferris is desperate because he's done the dirty in the beginning, and he wants to keep his little nose out of gaol. Desperate men make bad enemies."

"Lucknow makes me want to throw up, Sally growled. "I mean it."

"Yeah, sick perverted bastard," Pat agreed.

They didn't have time for further comment because Festerhaus came barrelling down the corridor towards them. "I want a report on the condition of the support system's musculature," he ordered. "Make sure it's up to scratch. I want a thorough massage of every muscle and joint from its neck down. Oh, and if you're thinking about stirring up rebellion, remember the consequences of being sacked are the same as violating your contract in the first place."

He strode off towards the biochemistry lab to make sure the next batch of neuroepithelial stem cells were ready for transplanting tomorrow, leaving a simmering group of support staff behind him. In retrospect it was a foolish and uncalled for provocation.

❋ ❋ ❋

The operation went seamlessly. A section of healthy cortical tissue was removed and replaced by what Lucknow called the witches brew of neural stem cells, utilising the same process which had been so spectacularly successful with the prefrontal cortex. The library was returned to recovery in the usual state of bruising around the face, and bandaging all over its head. The nurses, all of them, responded with meticulous post-operative care, largely because it was their only outlet for the feelings they were not supposed to have for it.

After a couple of months, Lucknow and Roberts treated the morning conference with the results.

"Well," Lucknow began, acknowledging the glare from Gilead with a smile, "you'll all be glad to know our support system doesn't want to bunny hop around the ward. In fact it probably can't walk at all now, but of course that's not a problem, seeing as it's never going to walk anywhere before you cut its legs off—"

Roberts, watching Gilead about to explode, interrupted. "My learned clown is trying to say the new tissue is not connecting. It's not wiring itself into the existing motor cortex. The number of layers is wrong, too. It's not an olfactory cortex either. I don't know what's gone wrong, but we've missed the mark by a mile this time."

"What do you mean it won't be able to walk? You mean you've given the girl a disability? Deliberately?" Sally Brown's face was black with rage.

"Of course we didn't want to give her a disability," Gilead retorted, resorting to the personal pronoun in his anger. "We're trying to learn how to repair tissue, and this time we've got it wrong, like our first attempt with the frontal lobe. Why can't you see this? I've had enough of the irrationality you spew out over us all, Brown. You should be able to do better. You've had this explained any number of times."

Ross stood to his feet. Unlike Sally Brown his voice was measured and quiet, the rage he was feeling inside completely hidden. "Professors Gilead and Metzger, eminent doctors, can I make a plea for a small alteration in our research methodology? The problem we are encountering is the same as before, although nothing as gross as an olfactory cortex has been produced. It is a problem with differentiation. As we are using the same method, the problem must lie with the motor neurons not expressing the correct environmental signals to allow our neural stem cells to form the correct neurons. As you know there are numerous ways to accomplish this, and without some better direction, we put our tissue library in unnecessary risk. We have a good sample of her... its.. motor cortex in vitro in the lab. Why not experiment on this until we have the right expression method, then introduce our NSC's?"

"I disagree with Ross on just about every moral issue he raises," Metzger said, "but in this case I believe his suggestion is worthy of merit. We always take some risk with the library when we open it. There is always the possibility of infection, or some other factor. I vote we use the in vitro approach in the short term. We can always harvest more tissue if we need to. When we get the method right we can replace it."

"I concur. What about you, Jan, Lavro?" Gilead asked, frowning.

Both men nodded their heads in agreement. The meeting broke up shortly afterwards, the support team feeling an almost palpable sense of relief.
For the next six weeks the geneticists and neurologists worked on the problem in vitro without resolving it at all. The more unsuccessful they

were, the more Gilead shied away from further surgery. No, he would not open the library on a whim. When they had solved the problem, and only then would he consider a further NSC implant, and he rejected Metzger's suggestion they harvest more motor area tissue.

Over those six weeks the tissue library began to grow a covering of beautiful dark brown curly hair, and with the constant attention of two nutritionists, three physiotherapists and ten nurses, began to look more and more like a beautiful young woman and less and less like the support system she was meant to be.

Cassie Clements, brushing her curly hair with gentle strokes one evening before she went off duty, was surprised to see Professor Gilead walk through the bio airlock into the ward. She stopped and rather nervously tucked the brush under the pillow. There was probably some rule against brushing a tissue library's hair, but she didn't care, she'd made her look very pretty.

"Good evening Professor Gilead," she stammered. "I was—"

"It's alright, Cassie. Please continue. I had no idea she had grown that much hair. You've made her very comfortable. Thank you."

Cassie didn't miss the personal pronoun.

"I'm sorry if I did something wrong... I just wanted to make her... she's a beautiful young woman, isn't she?"

Cassie knew it was verboten heresy to speak like that, especially to Gilead, but she was a perceptive member of her sex. There was something in the Professor's manner which told her, in the mysterious language which women read so well when they look at men, that her heretical comment would not initiate a tirade of censure, and it didn't.

"Yes, she is," Gilead said quietly. "I can see by the way you've been doing her hair that you care for her a great deal."

"I do, as a matter of fact." It was dangerous to say more, and Cassie, for all her training, could feel tears welling up in her eyes. She turned away, took her handkerchief out of her pocket and blew her nose. "I'm sorry. Must be the dry air in here."

"Perhaps. I'm grateful for your care, Cassie. No, I'm not patronising you. I am truly grateful. Without love we become less than human. You think of me as a ghoul and I don't blame you. I'm a man who tries to love too, but I do it in a different way."

"I... I don't know what to say, Professor. I think I'm too attached to Libby to be able to accommodate your kind of love towards her."

"Libby?" Gilead raised his eyebrows.

"That's what we nurses call the tissue library," Cassie stammered. "I've said too much. I'm tired. I should be going now. Please don't take it out on the others, it's all my fault."

"I cannot see how you are guilty of anything other than carrying out your role with dedication and – love. However you do it is fine with me. Please, go and have a rest. I think I would like to spend a little more time with ... Libby, as you call her."

Cassie thanked him and went through the air lock quickly. This was a side of Professor Gilead she had not seen and didn't know how to take at all. For half a second she wondered just why the man would want to spend time alone beside the beautiful young woman, and reproved herself for the thought. The Professor might be a ghoul of sorts, but he wasn't a pervert.

Gilead walked over to the corner of the room, brought back a chair, placed it down beside the bed and sat down on it. Yes, Cassie Clements had spoken the truth. Libby was a beautiful young woman. He could imagine her with her eyes open, brown eyes. He knew the colour, because he had lifted the lids and examined them for traces of retinal bleeding. How very well he could understand the feelings of his support staff. Perhaps he should instruct them to shave her hair off. No, it was good for them to have an outlet for their feelings. He stared at her again,

314

a young woman with a new mind, marred only by the healthy tissue he had cut from her motor cortex. Still, the problem would be solved, more tissue would be taken if needs be. Yet even as he thought the words he felt a sudden unwillingness to carry them out.

A young woman with a new unpolluted mind, a new spirit unsoiled, teachable, probably very intelligent if the number of sulci[3] in the new frontal lobes had anything to do with it. A creature with a mind of his making. What could she be capable of? Libby? A cheap epithet for library? Never. He gazed at the serene sleeping face, a princess waiting only for a single kiss to wake her. Odette, she was Odette, the Swan Queen, the one whom he had freed from Von Rothbart's curse, who could return to her human form and shed beauty and light into the world.

Would she love her liberator? It was love he craved, not sex. A daughter not a mistress, who would allow him to teach her, show her how to use her new mind, allow it to inform her heart, allow her heart to call a fresh springtime of understanding into a world beset with so much unnecessary sorrow.

A new mind, freed from the burden of being a soul.

But had he freed her? Was she not still bound in the form of a Swan, bound until his final word broke the spell? Did he dare? Should he dare? There was a quality in the vision before his eyes which he struggled to understand. Was it merely her beauty? No, something for which he had no name rose to summon his will onto a different course, something so compelling it was almost metaphysical, if there was such a thing, which of course there wasn't.

He stood, took one final look at the serene face, and walked towards the air lock, a deeply troubled man. He had always been able to apply his reason to every emotion, yet this one had defied him. His heart said what his mind disavowed. How had that happened?

---

[3] sulci, cortical folds. The average human cortex, if spread out, would cover over a square metre.

He didn't sleep well that night, for whenever he dozed off, pictures of Odette lying serene would rise before his mind.

Now she was speaking. "Wake me, my creator and teacher. Wake me, let me see your face. Let me be what you have made me. Don't take me apart. Allow me to become me, whole."

He saw his arm reaching out to remove the drip from her leg, pulling it out, watching her eyes open. She was reaching out for him, her face shining with joy, his own heart light as thistledown. Then suddenly he was staring at a his hands. Instead of removing the drip they had administered the fatal injection by mistake. He was ripping off the sheets, pressing his head to her chest, listening to the faltering beat of her heart, finally silent. He screamed out in agony of spirit and woke up, a lather of sweat covering his forehead and arms. He reached for his phone on top of the bedside table and clicked it on. Four thirty, and he felt so tired, so exhausted.

Further sleep was impossible. He staggered out into the kitchen and made himself a strong cup of tea. He could hear heavy rain beating against the window, and it was cold for the end of October. A strong gust of wind blew the rain harder against the glass. It would be a slow trip into Westmead this morning. Perhaps he should have a quick breakfast and set out. There was much he had to think through when he arrived.

CHAPTER 33

It was nine thirty five. Five men were gathered around the table at the back of the biochemistry lab, staring unhappily at the stained micrographs illuminated by the fluorescent screen on the wall nearby. Another test failed, and they were running out of tissue to test.

Metzger began the predictable discussion. "We've tried and failed again. We can only do this once, maybe twice more, and we will have to harvest more tissue. Perhaps we should sample some of the library's temporal lobe and see if we have any better luck with that, or the occipital. I can't see why we should allow the project to stall when we have other tissues to experiment with."

"I agree." Jan Yanac nodded. " Why not harvest some of them today? We could cut a slice or two out of its temporal lobes and see if our implantation method works as is. We might find the only problem lies with the motor cortex, although why it should still defies our explanations."

"It's time," Metzger said. "Shall I send for the nursing staff to prep the library? Have you noticed, its grown a lot of hair? Have to get that off first. Perhaps we should take a picture."

Gilead's dream kept interfering with his muddled thoughts. "I believe we should try those last two experiments before we open her head again." He said quietly.

"*Her* head? I beg your pardon?" Metzger was genuinely astonished. "Since when did our library acquire the status of a human being? I can distinctly remember your own words cautioning us against such thinking!"

"I know. Gentlemen, I have had a very bad night." Gilead wiped his arm across his forehead. "I beg you, set up our last *in vitro* tests and let us see if we can solve the problem. I admit I am loathe to arbitrarily slice pieces out of our Library just to see if we can replace them. You must remember we have been fortunate so far, but every time we open the skull we run a certain amount of risk. I will not condone further harvesting until we have at least performed our final tests."

"You begin to worry me, Isaac," Gerhardt frowned heavily. "You're not yourself. Perhaps it is best. Why don't you go home and get some rest? Take some sleeping pills from the pharmacy with you. We will carry on here until you get back tomorrow."

"Thank you Gerhardt. I believe I will take your advice."

Isaac Gilead left the room and returned to his office. There were a few urgent administrative matters he had to attend to, and then he would go home, catch up on the sleep he needed. The few matters took much longer than he had anticipated. A knock at the door brought him back to the realisation he had been there two and a half hours.

Ross entered, shut the door behind him, went over to the other chair and sat down. "I'm incredibly glad to find you in your office, Professor," he said in a worried voice. "I tried calling your mobile several times, but the call went straight through to your message bank. Your car isn't in the parking area either."

"No, I came very early, and the gate wouldn't open. Some new security rubbish probably, so I parked in the street," Gilead explained wearily. "I thought the walk across the bridge would clear my head, but it hasn't. I left my mobile at home, another symptom of my muddled mind. Can I help you?"

"That explains why Metzger believes you've gone home as you said you would." Ross took a deep breath. "I regret to inform you he has scheduled surgery on the library this afternoon. He intends to sample several areas of the cortex at the same time, and try NSC implants in all of them."

"What?" Gilead exclaimed, very much awake. He dropped the pen he was holding and stared at Ross in disbelief.

"I'm sorry to have to tell you," Ross continued. "I disagree totally with his approach. I thought you were in charge of this research unit."

"So did I," Gilead said. "When does the surgery begin?"

"In less than an hour. The nursing staff are distressed."

Gilead picked up the phone and rang the head nurse. "Ruth Garrard? I believe you have been given some instructions regarding the library? Yes? Have you shaved her head yet? No? Good. Gerhardt's instructions are countermanded as from this instant. You are to do nothing whatsoever to the library unless you receive instructions from me and me alone. Understand? It's alright, there's no need to thank me."

He put down the receiver. "I am grateful, Ross. Tell me, why have you broken ranks with the others to inform me? I can't think it will improve your standing with them."

"I'll be frank. I disagree with further surgery altogether," Ross sighed heavily.

"Are you a believer in God, David?"

"I am open to the possibility of a God. I am a believer in the soul, let us say. I believe there is more to a human being than the chemistry we observe. Regarding the mind as simply a giant computer seems to me to diminish our humanness. Computers make logical decisions, human beings make judgements. I think you may have forgotten that."

He paused to allow Gilead time to absorb his words. "We have done remarkable work here, work which needs to be shouted from the rooftops. I know more work is needed, but perhaps when the work which has been done is made public, other possibilities may come our way, ones we don't have to forge death certificates to obtain."

"And who would be our public advocate when this girl rises from the dead as it were?" Gilead replied bitterly. "You? Festerhaus? Not even Metzger would make a very good job of it. His temper would likely get us all thrown in gaol."

"The girl herself – Libby, as the support staff call her," Ross answered earnestly. "She's your perfect advocate. Can you imagine the impact that young woman would have on the world? She gets up and tells her story, says how everlastingly grateful she is for what has been done to her. She proves by her intelligence that the method is successful, extols our virtues to the mountain tops. You think anyone is going to be struck off or gaoled in the face of all that? ARG will get the publicity of a lifetime."

He spread his hands out towards Gilead in his characteristic imploring gesture. "What will happen if we continue our experiments, destroy her cortex, and finally have to do as Ferris and Lucknow keep on about, carve her organs out for sale, and dispose of the remains? With the girl gone we cannot prove our achievements."

He paused again, trying desperately to keep the passionate feelings out of his voice. "All it takes is one tiny slip up, someone notices something, asks the right question, and we're all heading for disgrace on every front, body snatching, vivisection, murder. You think the company will come to our rescue? They'll throw us to the wolves. No, my way is best, from all points of view. Once the world sees what we are capable of, I don't believe it will be at all difficult to obtain other people with brain damage in other areas who will be willing to put their lives in our hands."

Gilead sat silent for so long Ross wondered if he had heard him at all. Finally he spoke in a quiet, measured voice. "There's no such thing as a soul, David, you're wrong there. However, I believe you may be right about our advocate. If we had been able to solve the differentiation problem I would never have contemplated it. Now I've made up my mind, yes, I'm going to wake her up, and Gerhardt is going to be the second person to know."

He clenched his fists and brought them down hard on his desk. "How dare he take this research project out of my hands! He has brought this upon himself, and there is going to be some unpleasantness as a result."

Metzger was the second person to know. His surprise at seeing Gilead march straight into his room without knocking turned to anger when he learned his instructions had been countermanded, and molten rage when he learned of Gilead's intention to bring his tissue library back to full consciousness. The argument could be heard clearly up and down the length of the corridor. After five minutes every member of the support staff was listening in. Ferris was listening in too, and a cold sweat began to break out on his forehead. The door was flung open, and a furious Metzger marched past them all, swearing loudly to himself.

He turned to the joyful faces of the support staff lining the walls. "You stupid fools, he bellowed. "You think this is a good outcome? Damn and curse your hides. It will turn to your undoing if it's ever in my power. Now get out of my way."

He marched down the remainder of the corridor, opened the door which led into the imaging room and slammed it shut with a good deal more force than necessary. Sally Brown began to clap, and several others cheered.

❋ ❋ ❋

The meeting the following morning in the conference room was fire and brimstone from the start. Metzger had chosen to absent himself, and so battle lines were drawn with Yanac, Festerhaus, Ferris, Lucknow and Roberts on one side, and everybody else on the other. Max Hargraves sat by himself at the back of the room drinking black coffee and saying nothing at all. Lucknow demonstrated his superb skill with appalling language, and the support staff collectively hurled vitriolic defamation in reply. Festerhaus demanded the nurses defer to their betters in silence, and had to be rescued by Yanac when Pat Cornish went for him with a raised fork in her hand.

Gilead sat silently at the front, a sad and troubled expression on his face. When the antagonists had quietened down through sheer exhaustion, he stood up and resumed what he had tried to say in the beginning. "I accept full responsibility for my decision. I believe I have made it in the best interests of everyone here, including Libby herself. I have asked Ruth to remove the drip as soon as this meeting – if that is what you can call the appalling riot I have just had the misfortune to attend – comes to an end. I would ask all the support staff to keep a very close eye on our – patient – from that time on. I wish to be informed of any change, no matter how trivial. I would ask my colleagues for a quantum of understanding. We may have urgent need for your expertise at any time."

"Not me," Lucknow spat, "you can take your sex doll and do whatever you want to her without my help."

"Then, Doctor Lucknow, I would have to dismiss you," Gilead said, a furious expression on his face. "Please read your contract carefully. I am persuaded the consequences of your action would adversely affect your current lifestyle."

Lucknow responded by a long torrent of utterly foul language. He stood up, hurled his chair towards Gilead, and stormed out of the room.

Ruth took out the drip at exactly eleven fifteen a.m., and the team, even the geneticists, held their breath. What would wake up? A young woman with a functioning mind, or an animal without one? Throughout the day Gilead made hourly pilgrimages to her bedside, but there was no change whatsoever. One week later he ordered Lucknow and Roberts to monitor cortical activity, which they did with all the grace of a cornered hyena.

"There is a great deal of activity going on in there," Lucknow said, doing his best to keep a civil tongue in his head, "and the EEG is normal for someone sleeping. She's not coming to consciousness though. Perhaps you'll have to try something with your magic hands."

"Thank you, now get out," Gilead growled. You concur, Doctor Roberts?"

"I concur Herr Professor." Roberts and Lucknow left the room and slammed the door.

❄ ❄ ❄

A whole six weeks passed, and Libby showed no signs of returning to consciousness. Cassie Clements was used to Gilead appearing through the air lock half way through her evening shift. He would come over, smile, enquire politely concerning her health, her family, her day, and finally get round to the question he really wanted the answer to, although he knew it already.

"Has there been any change, Cassie?"

"No, Professor. Would you like to sit with her for a while?"

Cassie knew the answer to that question too. Out of courtesy she would leave the room, secure in the knowledge that this man cared every bit as much for Libby as she did. She would wait respectfully in the imaging lab, listening to music on her iPod until he came out, which could have been an hour later. She often wondered, did he talk to her? Watch her? Stroke her hair? She would have been right had she chosen all three.

This evening was different. There were tears in Gilead's eyes, and the sight of them shocked her profoundly. She knew instinctively they had reached the end of the road. The implants had failed, the girl would never wake up. Her own tears began streaming down her face, and she turned away to hide them.

Gilead reached out his hand and touched her arm gently. "I am so sorry too. I did... everything I knew how to do."

"I know you did," Cassie stammered. "I'm just sad, that's all."

There was nothing else to say. How different he was to the monster she had first supposed him to be. She left, turning finally as she passed through the air lock to see him sit down besides the sleeping girl.

"Why?" He spoke softly to her. "My Odette, why? I free you from the curse, yet you choose to remain a Swan. Have I betrayed you? Have I believed the lie, believed the mind I gave you would function and free you, when in fact it is nothing but a mass of tissue masquerading, an Odeil, a cruel imitation of the real. I have done everything in my power – to no avail. I have sacrificed my reputation, my leadership, all that was precious to me – gone. Yet you lie there, content to mock me. Am I your Siegfried destined to perish with you in the dark waters? But I will not."

He stood up, reached over the girl, ripped the sheet from her shoulders and shook her violently up and down against the bed. "Wake up. Wake up! Don't you know this is the final hour of grace? Soon it will run out. We will begin testing again, and you will disintegrate forever into the bodies of others. You could have been so much more. I offered you my love, my knowledge. You rejected them. How dare you! Enough. You've broken my heart and my life, but no, I will not drown for you, my Swan, and now, now you are lost forever."

He sat down heavily on the chair, cradled his head in his arms on the bed and wept.

It was December the twelfth.

That night Gilead phoned Metzger. He had little hope their relationship could be restored, and he was right. "Is that you, Gerhardt, my friend?"

"I am no friend of yours, Isaac," Metzger hissed down the phone. "You betrayed me. You betrayed all of us."

324

"Yes, I know that now," Gilead said sadly. "I have seen the folly of my ways. For an instant I came to believe in something irrational. Even now I cannot tell you why, but I repent. Is there no forgiveness for an old friend? Our lives go back a long way together."

"Old ways must part one day, Isaac. I can no longer trust you. You say you have repented, yet your repentance may not suit my taste. Exactly what have you repented of?"

"We have failed. The tissue library cannot achieve consciousness. I am going to reschedule our testing programme, and when it is over we will offer its working parts to others who need them. I am going to explain all at tomorrow's meeting, and I beg you to be there."

"I will be there," Metzger said, his voice like ice. "It's too late, Isaac. When I am betrayed I do not forgive. Goodnight."

Gilead put the phone down and wept.

CHAPTER 34

The day of the Storm

There was a sombre air in the conference room that morning, December the 13th. Some of the nursing staff were quietly weeping, the physiotherapists in an attitude of grief. Lucknow was lounging at the back of the room, his feet up on the table. He was drinking a bottle of beer, totally forbidden within the research facility. The other geneticists seemed far from friendly. Animosity or grief, Gilead thought as he stood and walked towards the white board. Who would have imagined it would come to this?

He cleared his throat. "Eminent colleagues," he began, then paused. "Where is Doctor Ferris?"

"Ferris is coming in later. Says he had a gut ache, probably from the thought of listening to you." Lucknow emptied the remainder of his beer down his throat and reached into his briefcase for another. Gilead's face fell even further.

He took a deep breath and continued. "I have made a serious error of judgement. I deceived myself into thinking we had succeeded. I allowed myself to believe in something metaphysical, irrational, and I have paid the price." He cleared his throat.

"I assumed the work we had done on our tissue library was successful, and I wanted to bask in our success," he cleared his throat again.

"Once again I was wrong. The implant has not been successful. The neurons have differentiated properly, but the new material has not connected properly to the old. When she came in here she was lacking some parts of her frontal lobes, now she is lacking all of them. We have also failed to produce any successful motor neurons. In short we have failed. The young woman who lies in our ward is further from recovery than when she came here, and it was already impossible then. She is, in every sense, dead, although she appears to be so fresh and alive. That is a tribute to the wonderful care she has been given throughout by our support staff who alone, out of all of us, deserve to be commended."

He paused and looked around him. There was no change, no fresh hint of sympathy. He went on. "I bitterly regret the insult I offered to my own eminent colleagues. I am sorry. I can say no more. The programme we began will now continue, with the added understanding that our young patient can never recover. All she can do is sacrifice the remainder of her life for the benefit of others. The magnitude of that benefit is now in your hands. We will begin sampling tomorrow. Ruth, I wonder if you would remove the central line from her leg? Tomorrow we will re-site a new line into the other leg, just to make sure no bacteria have accumulated on the surface of the old one. That is all. If you need me I will be in my office."

Gilead walked off the podium without another glance at his audience. There would be no change. His colleagues had lost respect for him, all except Ross, perhaps. Even though they might be more sympathetic, the support staff would hate what was to happen over the next months. He didn't blame them.

※ ※ ※

Ferris, as it transpired, wasn't suffering from any physical illness at all, if you don't count being stressed out of his mind. Since that terrible, irresponsible decision had come into effect he had been living on a knife edge. The research team had turned into a battlefield. Sooner or later someone would blow the gaff out of sheer spite, and they would all be heading for little rooms behind bars – or at least he would. He was the one who had procured the girl in the first place, and he knew ARG would throw him to the lions rather than accept the smallest responsibility for his actions. And what if the girl just happened to wake up? After such a long period in a coma she was hardly likely to be normal. With her mind fried by foreign genetics, she was much more likely to wake up a raving, violent lunatic, insane with rage. No one in the centre would be able to handle her. Before long she would be out on the street, causing havoc and drawing attention to what had been done to her. The Australian public would be screaming for blood before the day was done, his blood.

No, there was only one solution. After he had made arrangements with his odious but useful brother-in-law, he would return to the centre and deal with the tissue library. When everyone arrived the next day they would find his note. The support system had failed suddenly. He had gone into the ward, discovered that she had stopped breathing, and arranged instant disposal. They might not believe him, but they would stick to that story like glue, knowing the alternatives were so much more personally unpalatable. ARG would believe it too, in preference to any other explanation. The project would be shut down. Everyone would go back to their own lives without saying a word, and that would be that. Disposing of the girl would cost him big bucks, but anything would be cheap compared with the alternative.

His business with Fred Burgess had taken longer than he had expected, so he didn't arrive at the research centre until after four thirty p.m. The sky was black as night, and the street lamps were turning themselves on as he parked his car on the other side of the bridge, some distance from the building. The fewer people who knew when he had arrived, the better. Glancing up at the swirling blackness above him, he strode briskly across the bridge, and eventually into the foyer of the research centre. He slunk past Sharon behind the desk, and swiped his card through the reader, catching the lift up to the imaging lab. He was delighted to find the place so deserted. Gilead and the other geneticists had gone home. The only nurse on duty was Cassie Clements, keeping watch over her charge.

He waved to her as he came through the airlock. "Cassie, there's one hell of a storm brewing outside. Why don't you go home, and leave the night supervision to me? I've got a lot of work to do. Take the evening off, you deserve it."

"Doctor Ferris, are you sure that's okay? Professor Gilead—"

"I've checked with Gilead. Off you go. The tissue...err... Libby is in safe hands with me."

"That's very kind of you, Doctor Ferris," Cassie said happily. "It's my birthday, did you know? Now I'll be able to go out with my friends." She bounded away through the airlock.

Ferris went over to the girl. He noticed the library's hair had been beautifully combed. He ripped the sheet off, and was about to unplug the central line, only to find it had already been removed. How incredibly fortuitous. He extracted the urinary catheter, checked she was clean, and went back through the airlock into the pharmacy to prepare his lethal injection. At first he had planned to administer it before he wheeled her out into his car, but thought the better of it. If anything went wrong and someone saw him, the girl should still be breathing. Then he could concoct some plausible story about taking her for further tests. Once she was safely in the back seat, he would inject her and drive off. By the time he reached Northern Suburbs crematorium she would be dead and cold, ready for the fire. Perfect. He finished preparing the injection, took it into the ward and slipped it under the sheet.

Now to wait until the coast was clear and trundle her out, down one floor, along the corridor, and through the door leading to the emergency exit. On the other side of that door there was a long passage, which came out on the far side of the building. He would leave her there and go back for his car. It would be a simple matter to park it alongside the exit and transfer the girl to the back seat. At six p.m. he took the lift down to see how the land lay. Sharon was still on duty in the front office, absorbed with her mobile phone. An occasional person walked the lower corridor, and a ferocious storm was raging outside. All to the good. Fifteen more minutes passed. Sharon picked up her things and disappeared into the deluge beyond the front door.

MAC CUSITER

Now was the time.

He caught the lift back up to the ward, took the prepared note out of his pocket, and stuck it on the airlock door. He clicked off the safety brakes on the girl's bed, and began to wheel her out through the airlock, through the imaging room, down the lift. Poking his head out on the ground floor, he saw the coast was clear. He dragged the bed swiftly out of the lift, and began to push it towards the emergency door at the end of the corridor. If anyone saw him now... but no one did. He shoved the door ajar, and pushed the bed through. It swung shut behind him. Now he was in the clear. He began to push the bed towards the emergency exit, still quite a long way down the passage.

He had negotiated two thirds of this distance, when two unexpected events occurred almost simultaneously. First the lights went out, enveloping the corridor in total darkness. If emergency lighting had been installed, it wasn't working. Ferris kept pushing the bed along as fast as he dared, but then the next unexpected event occurred. The passageway to the emergency exit was straight, but it wasn't all on the same level. About twenty metres from the end there were half a dozen steps going down. Even if the lights were on, it was doubtful if Ferris would have seen them, pushing the bed from behind. In the dark they came as a complete surprise. The bed shot forward and bounced down the steps. Ferris fell flat on his face and knocked himself unconscious.

He came to consciousness a short time later, woozy and temporarily disorientated. He could feel blood trickling down the side of his face. What had happened? He waited until his head had more or less stopped spinning, felt around and found the steps. He edged himself down until he was on the flat again and began to move forward, running his hand along the wall and hoping there weren't any more steps. The first thing he collided with was the bed, lying on its side against the door at the end of the passage. Suddenly he remembered. There was a tiny torch attached to his key ring. He pulled it out of his pocket and squeezed it on, staring in shock at what its dim light revealed.

The girl was gone, the bed empty.

Not possible, he muttered to himself. He wrenched the sheet off. The injection had gone too, fallen out when the bed bumped down the stairs. That's what had happened to the girl too, he told himself, and very carefully began to make his way back to the steps. At the bottom of them he found the syringe, but the girl was nowhere to be seen. With an oath he tore down the corridor again, leant against the bar on the emergency door, and nearly fell out into the heaviest rain he had ever felt in his life. It was pitch black, save for the occasional flash of lightning, revealing a world awash with water. She had to be out here, but where? He had to wait until another lightning flash before starting off in search of her. His tiny torch was useless, hardly illuminating his own hands. As he watched it winked out, saturated by the torrent falling from the sky. Once again the lightning flashed, then once more. Suddenly he noticed something. A figure dressed in a white flapping gown was standing on the roadside, quite a long way from him. She was waving her arms around her head and moving in the strangest manner imaginable, twisting round and round relatively quickly for the slow progress she was making. Ferris smiled to himself. She was on the road, how convenient. All he had to do was go back for his car on the other side of the bridge, then drive back until he caught up with her. There was a wrench in the toolbox, quite perfect for knocking her out. Then he would bundle her into the back seat and inject her. The torrential rain would ensure nobody else was the wiser.

Relying on the flashes from the sky, he raced along the road, blinded by the driving rain. Now he had reached the bridge. There was a lot of water under his feet, too much. He was sliding, falling. He made a desperate grab at the railing as he shot out under it into the dark, raging torrent. The figure on the road paid no attention to his final, terrified scream. She turned up her head into the night, allowing the wonderful cool wetness to pour down her thirsty throat.

※ ※ ※

Gilead was woken at seven fifteen by an hysterical Ruth Garrard. She had come down from the nurses' quarters extremely late, because the power had gone off during the night and her alarm clock had malfunctioned. Coming into the ward she had found Libby gone, bed and all. A note from Ferris, stuck on the airlock with tape, had said something about the

Library going into convulsions during the night and finally dying. He had taken her for disposal. Gilead's head was swimming. It had been a frightful sleepless night. The storm had raged against his unit with such fury he had feared the windows would crack. Water was dripping down two of the walls. The power was still off, so it was a wonder his mobile was operating. Peering down to the road below at the unending rows of stationary cars, he realised it would take him forever to get to work even if he set out immediately. Ruth was hardly making sense in any case. How could Ferris have done all that so quickly? Foul play of some sort was at work. He told Ruth to contact Ross who lived much closer, rang off, and tried to call Metzger with absolutely no success. Some cell towers were functioning, most weren't. It was two p.m. before he managed to arrive at the research centre after a long gruelling drive. Metzger, Yanac and most of the support staff were already there when he arrived. He read Ferris' note and didn't believe a word of it. Where was the man?

He called a compulsory conference half an hour later. It was short and to the point.

"My ... friends," he began sorrowfully, "by now you will have heard that Libby is no longer with us. If Doctor Ferris is to be believed, she died last night, and he has taken it upon himself to dispose of her remains. I wish to emphasise none of this had anything to do with me. I first learned the news when Ruth rang me this morning. Whatever happened, we have lost our tissue library, which means the project has come to a dreadful and premature end. I am still trying to contact ARG, but I am sure they will agree with the course of action I now propose to take. You are all released from the project with full pay. If you take my advice you will all go home. Go home to where you were before we began, and if you can, try not to think too ill of me. I will remain for a short time assisting ARG to sell off the expensive equipment we have been using. It remains only for me to bid you farewell and good fortune. Maybe one day our paths will cross again. I hope so. It has been a privilege to work with most of you. I wish this chapter of our lives had turned out better than it has. Farewell."

Metzger left without so much as a 'good-bye', leading the other geneticists out the door.

Ross remained, came over and shook his hand. "You're a brilliant man, Professor Gilead. I shall always admire your courage. I would wish you a happy and fulfilling life."

Most of the support staff remained to thank him as well.

Cassie Clements was left sitting on a chair, her head in her hands, tears seeping through her fingers. Gilead approached her. "Thank you for your care of Libby," he said softly. "You are an excellent nurse, Ms. Clements, and—"

"It was all wrong," Cassie suddenly blurted out. "I'm so confused. She was such a beautiful young woman…" She stopped, blew her nose, and stood up, staring Gilead in the face. "I thought you were a monster," she said, "but you're not. You really loved her in your own way. I know you did. I'll always remember you differently from the others."

She kissed him on the neck and ran out of the room crying.

CHAPTER 35

Third year after the Storm

Isaac Gilead checked his way through front of house security at the Research Centre, and caught the restricted lift up to the first floor. He walked slowly across the corridor, and swiped his card into the reader on the biologically sealed door opposite. It opened with a soft hiss, and Gilead entered a world of technology any hospital would have given a great deal to own. The piece de resistance, a brand new six Tesla Functional Magnetic Resonance Imaging machine, stood in the far right hand corner next to its control booth. In the adjacent corner of the opposite wall, surrounded by a magnetic isolation cage, the latest Positron Emission Tomography unit hummed quietly. Next to that machine was a the lead lined room from which radioisotopes could be added to a wide range of molecules, depending on which sort of neural activity was being monitored.

On the other side of the door stood a conventional Computerised Axial Tomography machine. Another doorway to the right of the machines led to the two specialised biochemistry and genetics laboratories, recently refurbished with all their highly specialised gear. Further along the corridor which Gilead had crossed, lay the freshly painted offices for the technical staff, including the large conference room. The floor above would soon house the support staff that Metzger had chosen for the new project, nurses, technicians and nutritionists. All was quiet except for the faint muted purr of the cryogenics, and the soft hiss of triple filtered air blowing from the vents in the ceiling. No micro-organism from the outside world could enter here, and likewise, nothing created in here could venture by accident into the outside world. It had been a frenetic exercise to equip the new centre, but now all was in readiness.

Gilead stared at the doorway directly opposite him, the surgically clean space which would once again contain the single most important item in the whole research complex. Without it the entire centre, with all its extremely expensive technology and highly trained staff, was totally without purpose. Tissue library thirty, complete with its own support system, would be installed soon. In a fortnight's time staff would all arrive, both old and new, ready to continue the ground-breaking research begun some five years ago, five years which seemed like a day in some ways, like an age in others.

He turned and walked slowly out of the imaging lab, down past the empty offices to the conference room, also empty. He turned on the lights and sat down in a once familiar chair at the head of the large dark mahogany table. He shut his eyes. So familiar, so different. Soon he would be meeting with all those other colleagues as he had done on that first day five years ago, only this time he would not be in this old familiar chair. He would miss that chair, miss his familiar place as head of the team, miss it very much.

So many painful memories. He had never ever thought to be part of another tissue library project, yet here he was, invited by the very man he thought hated him forever. He heard a sound behind him and turned around to see Metzger enter the room.

He came over and held out his hand. "Isaak, Isaak, wie gut es ist, dass Sie nach so vielen Jahren zu sehen.[4] You haven't changed at all."

"I fear you exaggerate, Gerhardt my old friend. It is good to see you too. What do you think of our facilities?"

---

[4] Isaac, Isaac, how good it is to see you after so many years.

"The best, Isaac. I knew you would obtain the best. Now for the best news. I am going to acquire our new tissue library in a few days. By the end of the week the rest of the team will begin arriving, and in a fortnight's time we begin again."

"I am filled with gratitude, Gerhardt. I am trembling with excitement."

"You will certainly tremble with something," his old friend replied.

CHAPTER 36

J ames Hunt smiled abstractedly at the bearded customer. He ran his credit card through the reader, which obligingly produced the little piece of paper for the customer to sign. Hunt barely noticed. His mind was preoccupied with another matter, which had grown to such proportions it haunted his dreams as well as his days. He took the signed slip from the customer, and out of habit rather than thought, wished him a pleasant evening.

"What's pleasant about it?" the customer growled. "Have you seen what's outside? I've gotta drive home in that, while you sit on your arse wishing people a bloody good evening."

The customer grabbed the paper and headed out into the night, or what seemed to be night, even though it was only seven p.m. at the end of January. Gazing beyond the covered concrete apron of the petrol station, Hunt could see what he meant. Heavy rain bucketed down from an ink black sky. Even as he watched, small white balls of hail began to rain down onto the paved apron beyond the metal sails which covered the pumps. Drivers were pulling in one after another seeking their meagre shelter, two deep against every pump. Pity help the poor driver who actually wanted fuel. The hail was heavier now, the racket on the galvanised roof of the office deafening. On the street beyond the garage, motorists were pulling over into the curb, their vision reduced to zero. Now the white pebbles had graduated into full sized hailstones the size of golf balls. Hunt wondered just how many were caught in the gutters which drained the sails. If those blocked, the weight of ice building on top would bring down the sails. Those who had driven under them for shelter would be in far more danger than they had faced on the street. What a storm. Now the hail was lessening, only to be replaced by a tropical torrent of water streaming from the sky.

What a storm. What a... STORM!

Hunt smashed his fist onto the counter. Storm. What a bloody fool he'd been. The girl's name, Storm, so unusual. Why call her that? Because that was when she had arrived without any other name, on the night of the cyclone which hit Sydney just over three years ago, the same night Ferris had died. Suddenly he remembered something Patricia Fletcher had said. They were taking care of a patient who needed constant attention. A patient, why didn't he twig to it before? Three physiotherapists caring for *a* patient, singular. It wasn't the loss of Ferris which had cancelled whatever was going on there, it was their patient. They'd lost their lab rat, the raison d'étre of the whole project. Whatever they had been doing to her was so illegal, so unethical, they had scuttled like rats as soon as she was gone.

What to do now? Patricia Fletcher wasn't only afraid, she was distressed. Perhaps she had developed a fondness for the lab rat while she was treating her. A long shot, but then the only advances he had made on the story were from long shots. At that very instant the power failed, plunging the garage into total darkness. His shift was due to finish in an hour anyway. Well, tonight it would finish early. He opened the small safe under the counter, and emptied the cash drawers into it. He took the keys and a torch, went out under the sails which thankfully hadn't collapsed, and locked every pump. Half an hour later he was on the motorway heading north towards Gosford. An hour after that he arrived at the cream brick house in Maiden's Brush Road and rang the bell.

Tony Fletcher answered, recognised Hunt, and tried to shut the door in his face. Hunt jammed his foot against the wood, pushed a startled Tony out of the way and stepped into the hall.

"I've come for some answers," he growled. "Try to shove me out and I'll be back with Gosford police. You won't enjoy what happens next. I'm trying to save a woman's life, and your wife is going to help me."

It was pure bluff, but effective. The colour drained from Tony's face. Patricia, who had arrived in the hallway in time to hear Hunt's little piece of fantasy, gave a horrified cry and looked as though she was going to faint. Hunt was quick to capitalise on his advantage. He strode towards Patricia, pulling the photo of Storm, Village Artist, out of his pocket. He shoved it into her face. "Was this the patient?"

The effect was better than expected. Patricia Fletcher collapsed into his arms, rather complicating matters. Tony Fletcher leapt forward. Hunt carefully transferred the unconscious woman into her husband's arms, which prevented the man from kicking him into next week, the message clearly written on his face. Tony carried his wife into the living room rather than the bedroom, which was promising of further interaction. By the time he had placed her carefully on the lounge she was wide awake and very vocal.

"Libby. Libby! No. It can't be Libby. Oh merciful God, say it is. How? How is this possible? Oh Libby."

Tears were streaming down her face. Hunt could only guess who Libby was, but the overall message was clear enough.

"Tell me the whole story," he urged. "This girl is in danger, and as far as I know you are her only help."

Patricia Fletcher eyed Hunt up and down as though she didn't believe a word of it. Her first question threw him. "Libby died. She wouldn't wake up. Tell me, why should I believe a damn thing you say?"

Hunt could see there was no way to bypass the question if he was to learn anymore, so he gave her as detailed an answer as he could. He decided it would be better not to add fabrication to fact, and left out all the stuff about saving her life. It was well that he did.

Patricia turned sorrowfully towards her husband. "Tony, I'm so sorry. I'm so sorry. I'm going to tell him. I know what's likely to happen, but I can't live with myself if anything happens to Libby. If those swine ever learn she's alive they'll want her back. I just couldn't cope with ... " She burst into tears again.

Tony sat beside her and put his arm around her back. "You don't have to say anything to this self-serving piece of garbage."

"But I do," Patricia sobbed. "I loved Libby. Tell me, Mr... James, isn't it? Is she really conscious? I beg you, I really beg you not to lie to me."

"See for yourself," Hunt answered. "This is a cutting out of the Northern Voice regional newspaper. If you don't believe me, check it out on line."

"You say she's an artist? Can she talk? Is she intellectually disabled?"

"Not in the least. She's an incredibly gifted artist. As well as that, she did her Higher School Certificate last year and came eighth in the state. Here." Hunt produced the page from the Sydney Morning Herald. "She goes under the name of Helen Craig as I told you."

Patricia took the paper from his hand. She stared at the name and once again burst into uncontrollable sobbing, punctuated with the phrase "thank God, oh thank God" over and over again. Hunt was relieved to see the expression on her husband's face had changed from murder to confusion.

Eventually the sobbing stopped. Patricia blew her nose hard on her husband's handkerchief. "Can she walk properly?" she asked suddenly.

Hunt stared at the woman. "No, she's a cripple. What on earth made you ask that?"

"The bastards!" Patricia exploded. "Well, Mr. James, I'll tell you all you want to know. If it ever gets back to Amity-Rand Genetics they'll destroy our lives. You should know that."

"If this is what I think it is, Amity-Rand Genetics will be running for cover if the story goes public," Hunt assured her. "It's your best defence, besides helping Libby, as you call her. Please, tell me what happened in there."

Patricia Fletcher told him. She poured out all her fierce, passionate hatred for Gilead and the other geneticists. She recounted the horror of that last meeting when they had learned Libby was beyond cure, and would eventually be killed and have her organs sold off. She described the relief they felt when they had learned she had suddenly died, bringing the project to a grinding, blessed stop.

"It was all lies, all lies," she stammered. "Libby was just a tissue library for them to play around in. She was a young woman to all the rest of us. Why say she was dead? What happened to Ferris? I hope they all rot in gaol for the rest of their lives," she added vehemently.

"I can't answer your questions – yet," Hunt said. "You have to admit their work was an incredible success – except the last bit. The young woman's brilliant."

"I suppose so," Patricia sniffed. "Why tell us different? Gilead wanted to wake her up, but she wouldn't."

"How could they know their experiments had been successful, if she didn't wake up?" Hunt suggested. "Perhaps they thought it had all gone wrong." Hunt ran his hand through his hair, his mind processing the possibilities. "I'm going to see this girl tomorrow, because apart from all I've learned tonight, I know who she actually is, or I'm pretty sure of it. I promise not to reveal my sources, but as I said, the safest way is to make this whole sorry business public knowledge. ARG won't dare try anything nasty after that."

"I hope you're right, Mr. James," Patricia said, emotion surging through her voice. "I want you to know I'm grateful. You've told me Libby is alive, and I want to jump up and down for joy and thank God for it. She was such a beautiful young woman. We all became so fond of her."

A smile caressed Patricia's face for the first time ever. Tony resembled a stunned mullet, staring at his wife as if she had grown another head.

Time to leave, Hunt thought, and with a brief "thank you, I'll see myself out," he stood up and made his way down the corridor and out the front door. What a story. He'd won the jackpot. No more Mr. Garage Attendant after this. He reached into his pocket and clicked off the small recorder, although he hardly needed it. The details of Patricia's confession burned clearly into his brain. He remembered her words "if they find out she's alive they'll want her back." Yes, they would. Tissue libraries who were officially dead and cremated weren't all that easy to come by. Now to write up his notes and visit the girl, tell her carers, the Craigs, just what had gone on. Time they were in the loop. He hardly slept that night.

❋ ❋ ❋

Ellen Craig was bored. Peter had driven Storm to the Village for her Saturday D&C, draw and collect, the title she had bestowed upon Storm's artistic enterprise much to her family's disgust. He had returned home and gone into his bedroom to study. Basa was out shopping, and Andrew was attending to a patient or two in the surgery. The book she had been reading was boring, the plot so predictable, the hero a mindless jerk. She was about to throw it onto the pile on her bedroom floor which had grown considerably since she began to enjoy books, when the doorbell rang. Ellen wrapped her dressing gown around her. In complete disregard of her mother, who told her she was never to answer the door dressed like that, she walked down the corridor and answered it. A man stood in the doorway.

"Hello," Ellen said, "I remember you. You bought a glass of awful lemonade and one of Helen's pictures."

"I did," Hunt smiled at her. "You have an excellent memory, Miss Ellen Craig. I wonder if I might have a word with Helen. Is she available?"

"And you would be?"

"Sorry, James Hunt. I'm a freelance reporter. Please don't be alarmed. I have some news your ... ah... sister will want to hear."

The expression on Ellen's face told Hunt he was treading on dangerous ground. He could see her hand gripping the door, and knew it would be closing in his face any second. "Please," he said earnestly, "I don't want to alarm you, but there's a real possibility she might be in danger. Please. I just want to talk to her. It's very important."

"She hates publicity," Ellen said sharply. "Swear you're not going to take her picture."

"Okay, now can I speak to her?" Hunt insisted. "You can listen in if you're worried."

He had said the right thing at last. Ellen relaxed her grip on the door. "She's where she always is on Saturday mornings, at the Village, fleecing stuck up people who want portraits of themselves hanging on the wall."

"Thanks. See you soon. Ciao."

Ellen watched Hunt sprinting off towards his car with misgivings. Had she said too much? She ran back to the bedroom, threw on the essentials, and shot down the corridor towards the surgery. There was something bad going on here, and Dad ought to know. The doorbell rang just before she reached the surgery door. What to do? Perhaps this James Hunt was back. She had better find out. Running down the corridor she flung open the front door, prepared to do battle. Her face lit up in surprise. "Uncle Brian."

"Hello, Ellen. Is Dad in? I wanted to—"

"The name James Hunt mean anything to you?"

The smile on Brian Craig's face froze. "How do you know that name?"

"He was here a minute ago, wanting to speak to Storm. Shot off to the Village like the devil was after him. There's something bad going on."

343

"I'll check on Storm," Brian said hurriedly. "Tell Dad will you? Probably nothing to worry about, so don't go making up any end-of-the-world stories. See you soon, Ellen."

Uncle Brian flew back to his car as if the same devil had found another target. *Something is really going on*, Ellen thought to herself. The morning had suddenly improved enormously.

❄ ❄ ❄

The usual crowd was waiting when Storm arrived carrying her portable easel and drawing gear. It was incredibly hot that morning. She parked her crutches against the glass supermarket front, waved to Matthew on the other side, and wiped her face with a handkerchief. She stood the easel up and placed the wad of A2 drawing paper in the tray. Unslinging her backpack with all her drawing paraphernalia, she began to hand out tickets to her customers, who had already gathered despite the heat. She had long since discovered this was the best way of doing business, giving everyone a ticket and sticking a large piece of cardboard with her current client number up on top of the easel. It saved people waiting, and they could see from a distance how she was going.

Her first subject was a woman in her early forties who had dressed for the occasion. Storm, resisting the temptation to diminish the assets the woman so obviously wished to include in the portrait, subtly morphed them into film star proportions. A one hundred dollar note fluttered into her ice cream container, proof positive she had read her subject's thoughts accurately enough. Then there were three restless children held steady by their harassed mother, who kept repeating her apologies every time they complained. They wanted ice cream, chips, toys, lemonade. They were hot, they wanted to go to the toilet, had to go to the toilet. Storm was glad to see the last of them. Two hundred dollar notes fluttered into her container, fifty more than necessary, and when she proffered change the young mother shook her head and whisked the brats away as fast as she could.

The next client was an older gentleman. He sat down in the seat, opened a cooler bag and proffered her a bottle of lemonade.

344

"It's so hot, young lady," he said. "I thought you might need a drink, especially after those children. You showed remarkable patience."

"Thank you." Storm took the bottle and had a long drink. It was cold and refreshing. Now to begin work. The man had an interesting face, wise, lined with many years of hardship perhaps. It was the eyes which drew her attention, eyes which seemed in some indefinable way to display a cruelty at variance with the rest of his countenance, an implacable determination, careless of others. She was reading too much, and yet those eyes began to frighten her. *Oh!* She thought suddenly, *my tummy is giving me trouble. Must have eaten breakfast too fast or something. Oh, now it's worse.*

"Oh." She gave an audible groan and doubled up in pain.

The older gentleman looked startled. "My dear young woman, what seems to be the matter?"

"My tummy," Storm groaned. "Oh. I've got awful cramps. I think I'm going to be sick. You'll have to excuse me… OH!. She reached for her crutches, but by now her head was swimming so badly she could hardly thrust her arms into the collars.

"My dear, you are far from well," the older gentleman said. "I'm a doctor by profession. I insist in accompanying you to the toilet. When you've finished throwing up, I'll drive you home. It could be this heat, you know."

Storm was in no condition to refuse. Somehow she managed to slip into her crutches and make her way around to where the public toilets were, reaching the side of the building before she threw up all over the ground. Now she was feeling so ill her legs could no longer hold her, and she slid down against the wall.

The older man was watching her, a curious expression on his face. "My dear," he said, smiling. "I have a small injection here which will make you feel better. In fact, you'll never have to bother about those crutches again."

Storm stared into his face, horrified. She saw him withdraw a syringe from his pocket, felt him grab her arm and pull it towards him. Suddenly she knew the darkness had found her. She read her death in his eyes, and tried to cry out in terror, but the world was beginning to lose its solidity, swimming around in front of her eyes, growing darker. She collapsed against the side of the toilet block.

"How convenient," Metzger said to himself, and wrenching her arm up towards him, stuck the needle point into her smooth skin.

❋ ❋ ❋

Hunt parked his car in one of the few spots available at the Village, got out and sprinted towards the shopping complex. His eyes searched the Saturday morning crowd for any sight of Storm. Nothing, damn it. Where was she? Suddenly he spied the easel, set up in the shade of the awning which ran the length of the supermarket. He made his way over towards it. A number of people were milling around the area. One woman was sitting in what was obviously the artist's portrait chair.

He went up and spoke to her. "Hi, I'm trying to find the young artist. Have you seen her?"

"She was here a minute ago drawing an older man," the woman said. "I was next in line. He gave her some lemonade, and she started to draw him, but suddenly she said she felt ill and had to go to the toilet around the corner there. The gentleman said he was a doctor and went with her. She should be back in a minute."

A sudden fear gripped Hunt's heart. "What did he look like, this gentleman?"

The woman stared at him as though he was utterly stupid. "Like that," she said, and pointed to the drawing. Hunt turned round and stared. The portrait wasn't finished, but it was recognisable enough.

"Bloody hell, Metzger!" He shouted.

"What are you doing here, Hunt?" Brian Craig was running towards him. "Where's my niece?"

"In one shitload of trouble," Hunt yelled, and bounded away with Craig following hot on his heels. They tore around the side of the building heading for the toilet block.

A dreadful sight met their eyes. Storm was slumped against the wall surrounded by vomit. As he watched, Metzger snatched her arm, drawing it up towards the syringe in his other hand. The needle penetrated her skin. Hunt realised he wasn't going to make it before the contents of that syringe had been emptied into her arm. Snatching his mobile phone from his pocket, he hurled it towards Metzger. It was a good shot. Out of the corner of his eye Metzger saw it coming, and jerked his syringe-holding arm up to protect his face. The phone glanced of his forearm, and the syringe flew off onto the pavement. He stared uncomprehending at the two men racing towards him. For a second he seemed paralysed with indecision, then he took off as fast as he could run. Another man, who Hunt recognised as Jan Yanac, emerged from the men's toilet, assessed the situation and disappeared back in again.

"Get him!" Hunt bellowed at the top of his voice. "There's another one in the dunny."

Sliding down beside the unconscious girl, he lifted her head up from where it had fallen in the vomit on the ground, and let it rest against his shoulder. His heart was seething with anger. Seconds too late. Damn Metzger to hell. He gazed at her beautiful face and swore softly and long. If she died he was going to kill him, kill him with his bare hands. He looked up. Brian was returning with the prisoner, held by the arm in a vicious grip.

Metzger wore an arrogant smile all over his face. "This is all a dreadful mistake," he purred. "I'm a qualified doctor, a professor of neurology, in fact. The young woman was taken ill. On the way to the toilet she vomited and collapsed. I was alarmed, so I was about to give her an injection which would have settled her stomach and made her feel better."

Hunt sprang up from the wall, grabbed the syringe which was still lying on the footpath, and plunged the needle all the way into Metzger's neck.

"Let go, Craig," he shouted. "There's another of the swine in the Men's dunny. Can you lock him in? Make one twitch, Metzger," he snarled, "and this harmless stuff goes straight into your carotid artery."

"No! No, I beg you." Metzger's voice was almost a scream.

Brian, somewhat stunned by the turn of events, released Metzger and raced to the men's toilet. He swung the metal door shut and clipped a pair of handcuffs around the bars to keep it that way. Metzger had gone a funny shade of pale, and beads of sweat were forming on his terrified face.

Brian came up close to the terrified man. "What's in the syringe?" he snarled. "I'm going to count to three, and then my friend Mr. Hunt is going to squeeze. You don't mind, do you, Mr. Hunt?"

"My pleasure. Twitch a muscle, Metzger, and you get it anyway."

Metzger stood as still as a terrified tree trunk. He said some long name which Brian wrote down on his arm.

"And while we're at it," Hunt added, "what was in the lemonade?"

"I... don't know what you're talking about," Metzger stammered.

"Here it comes. Enjoy." Hunt gripped Metzger viciously around the shoulder and wiggled the syringe.

Metzger spouted another name which Brian wrote down next to the first one.

"Get backup," Hunt snapped. "Doctor Metzger is going to stand here like a telegraph pole."

Brian fished out his mobile phone and rang a number. "What would you like to charge him with?"

"Abduction and attempted murder. Okay?" Hunt wiggled the syringe.

"Fine with me," Brian grimaced. "And the one who's trying to rattle his way out of the dunny?"

"Accessory to both counts."

"Sounds good."

By now a small crowd of horrified shoppers had come belting around the corner. They took one look at Hunt holding a syringe in another man's neck, and screeched to a grinding halt, standing at a distance. Matthew from the supermarket pushed through the crowd and sat down against the wall next to Storm. He lifted the unconscious girl's head up from the pavement where it had fallen again and held it against his own shoulder, terribly worried and furious at the same time. Within five minutes the wail of police sirens could be heard in the background. A short time later Brian's mate Daniel Lucas with a few other officers came charging round the corner. They handcuffed Metzger and Yanac, then escorted them away. In the days which followed their initial incarceration, Yanac, trying to sidestep the inevitable, divulged everything, much to Metzger's disgust.

Hunt turned to Craig. "Can we get her to hospital on siren?"

"We take her to my brother," Craig answered. "He's a good doctor. See what he says. Come on."

The two men lifted Storm's unconscious body and ran with her to the police car. Brian leapt into the driver's seat and they took off under siren, lights flashing.

It was Ellen who noticed them first, Ellen who had deliberately stayed out the front of the house in anticipation of forthcoming events. She saw the police car arrive under siren, slew across the traffic, bounce into the driveway and screech to a stop. Uncle Brian leapt out and ran towards her. James Hunt went for the rear passenger door, opened it and lifted an unconscious Storm out in his arms. Ellen stood with her mouth open and her eyes wide as saucers.

"Get Dad. Hurry girl," Brian yelled at her.

Ellen flew inside and emerged with Andrew and Basa, who had returned from shopping. Peter and Ellen brought up the rear.

Andrew ran to Hunt and pulled Storm into his own arms. "What happened?" he cried.

"She's been poisoned, and possibly injected with some toxin," Brian said. "I've got the names."

Andrew ran into the surgery. Basa read the information from Brian's proffered arm and said several words in Hungarian with a very pale face.

"Dear God," she muttered as she sped after her husband, "if any of that's in her system we're in terrible trouble."

The door of the surgery slammed shut leaving four very worried people outside.

Peter was the first to remember his manners. "Please come in, Mr. Hunt. Ellen and I would like to know what happened at the Village. I didn't realise you were working with Uncle Brian."

"I wasn't," Hunt grimaced. "Let's just say our paths crossed at a most opportune time."

Inside the surgery Andrew had laid Storm down on the examination table. Basa was taking her blood pressure, measuring her pulse, both of them hoping desperately that either none or very little of the injection had found its mark.

"She'll go into a coma," Basa stammered, tears streaming down her face. "How could this have happened? God, what were you thinking of?"

Andrew shook his head and administered an injection to counteract the effects of the lemonade. He gripped his wife's arm, knowing how frightened she felt. "Courage, my love," he said softly. "All we can do is—"

"Daddy?" A soft, frightened little voice.

Two heads swung round to the figure on the bed. Her eyes were open, staring upwards.

Andrew gave a great cry and gathered her into his arms. "Oh, Storm, Storm my darling girl. We thought—"

"Daddy! How did I get here? He was going to... to... "

She burst into a fit of uncontrollable sobbing, clinging both to Andrew and Basa at the same time. At first she couldn't say anything, and she was shaking so badly Basa thought a sedative might be in order, but was unwilling to give it to her in case it interacted with the other toxin in her system. Eventually the sobbing died down a little, and Basa was able to answer her question.

"Uncle Brian and a man called James Hunt brought you back in the police car. That's all I know. You're safe now, darling. I don't think he managed to get any of that terrible stuff into you. It's alright, darling, it's alright."

By this time Storm was sitting on the edge of the examination table, her face buried in Andrew's chest, her arms around him. Basa opened the surgery door to the anxious faces on the other side. She told them Storm was going to be okay, and asked Ellen to bring her another set of clothes. Half an hour later Andrew carried her into the house, lowered her carefully on the lounge and sat down beside her. Basa sat down on the other side, Ellen at her feet on the floor. Peter, coming in from the kitchen with Hunt and Brian, stood over near the television looking worried and miserable, while the two gentlemen occupied the remaining chairs.

"Now," Andrew said in a worried voice, "perhaps someone will be good enough to tell us what all this is about."

Brian nodded towards Hunt. "I think James ought to be the one to do that. He's been on the ball a lot better than we have. If it wasn't for him, Storm would be—" He stopped suddenly.

"Dead," Storm said softly. "Worse than dead. Thank you, James. You know about my past, don't you? Do you know my real name?"

"Yes, I think I do," Hunt replied softly. "Are you sure you're up to it, Miss Storm? You've had a terribly close call, you know. Might be better later."

"No, now, please. I have to face it sometime. Am I a terrible person? A... a criminal?"

"Of course you're not," Basa interjected passionately.

"No, of course you're not," Hunt echoed. "Well here goes. Your real name is Felicity Demarra, the supposedly deceased daughter of Rachel Demarra, the actress."

Storm's pretty face crumpled up. Tears began to stream down, and she turned into Basa's breast, sobbing fit to break every heart in the room. Basa wrapped her arms around the girl. James was mortified. This was hardly the reaction he had expected or wanted to produce. He felt utterly wretched.

"No, no, no." Muffled words came from the sobbing girl. "Not that woman. No. I'm so ashamed. No."

"Storm, darling, it doesn't matter who your mother is. You're still our Storm, and we love you, we'll always love you," Basa comforted, holding her tightly and rubbing her back with her hand.

"It doesn't make any difference," Andrew assured her. "None. Your family is here, Storm. Like Mum says, we love you, we'll always—"

"Won't want me now... a disgrace ... can't face it... Oh, I wish I'd ... died." The words were punctuated with heartfelt sobbing.

Peter came over slowly, and kneeling down besides the distraught girl, reached out and rested his cool hand gently on her neck. He felt a shiver run through her body. Something about his touch brought a lull to the sobbing.

"Storm, please hear me." He waited until she was completely quiet then went on. "Storm, does Jesus love you?"

There was a pause, and then, muffled and soft, a reply. "Yes."

"And do you think for a single moment Jesus didn't know who you were? That He hasn't been the one taking care of you, bringing you to us, surrounding you with our love and His?"

There was silence.

"Don't you remember," Peter continued softly, "He was the one who set you free from the darkness in the first place, brought you here. He was the one who rescued you from the darkness today. Why do you suppose He did that? Because he wants you to live and love Him, Storm. You can't wish away the gift without wishing away the Giver."

For two interminable minutes there was absolutely no response. Then slowly, deliberately, Storm turned her head and stared at him in silence, as if she was measuring the words he had spoken. Her eyes read the familiar message written so plainly on his face, searching for the slightest hint of a change. There was none. More minutes passed in the total silence of the crowded room. Finally, without another word, she lay back against the sofa, Basa's arm still round her shoulder.

"Tell me the rest," she said.

Hunt did, and long was the telling, his audience speechless, hanging on every word. Basa turned ashen as Hunt told her about tissue library twenty nine, her eyes filled with horror. Andrew seemed deeply shocked, and gathered Storm's cold hands into his own, held them tight. Brian wore a grim expression which told the whole world he had scores to settle. Ellen had literally wrapped herself around Storm's legs, her eyes wide and frightened at the terrible images which Hunt's words were generating in her mind. Peter stood by the television away from the rest, deep in his own private thoughts and fears.

Finally Hunt stopped, but the silence remained.

Eventually Brian cleared his throat. "Brilliant. Simply brilliant. I've got to hand it to you, James. We've been chasing this thing ourselves right up to the Commissioner level, but we haven't made the progress you have. We knew ARG was starting up again, but that's about all we knew. I think we've got enough together to put Metzger and his mates where they belong, but what about Storm's real identity? Without that, ARG can wiggle out on the basis of circumstantial evidence. I take it you could convince a jury she's Felicity Dem—" He stopped suddenly again, not wishing to precipitate another burst of sobbing.

"Well, that's just the point," Hunt said slowly, "I can't, but I'm absolutely sure I'm right. For starters, Storm is the splitting image of her mother."

Storm sat up on the lounge, her eyes blazing. "Of course James is right. It all makes perfect sense. Isn't there any way to prove it? Surely there must be."

"Well," Hunt said, "I've been studying Rachel Demarra pretty closely. I think there might have been a way, but it relied on something I don't think Storm can do. She's a cripple, and my plan would require her to walk."

"I *can* walk," Storm protested. "I can't walk very well, and I'm slow, and unsteady, and it takes heaps of concentration. Tell me what you want me to do, James. If I have to walk, I'll walk. I'll walk if it's the last thing I do. Anything. Don't you understand? I want my name back. Even if it's one I really don't like, it's better than not having a name at all."

There was a note of fierce determination in Storm's voice, and her blazing eyes brooked no argument to the contrary.

Andrew read those eyes. He nodded to Hunt. "Okay, if it doesn't put Storm in the slightest danger, and I mean the slightest danger, we're with you. Tell us what you want us to do."

Hunt did.

Half an hour later Andrew rang Barrister Rowland Harris. "I'm about to call in that favour," he said.

CHAPTER 37

Chikkie Manners painted another toenail and waved her hand around her foot to help the varnish dry. Her room at the Sydney Hilton was far from her liking. All she could see of the harbour was a tiny bit of the Opera House, and a long row of apartments nearby which reminded her of a cheap oversized toast rack. How on Earth such a tasteless structure had been built so close to an iconic work of art she had no idea.

Rachel Demarra had chosen her as personal assistant some two years ago, in what subsequently proved to be a mutually beneficial arrangement. To those she wished to impress, manipulate or seduce, Chikkie Manners was Rachel's self-effacing advocate and polite facilitator, a role she endured without protest. To those the actress loathed, or for whatever reason didn't wish to see, she was an effective firewall, a role Chikkie enjoyed very much. Such people afforded her the opportunity to practice her acerbic wit and belittling, hostile manner. She accomplished this with such skill she became known by a rather derogatory nickname, which sounded quite similar to her real one. Fortunately for Chikkie there were far more folk in the latter category, so her life was more enjoyment than endurance. Added to these excellent qualifications was her rat cunning ability to accurately distinguish between the two classes without always having to be told.

James Hunt was one of the rare occasions on which she wasn't quite sure. Freelance reporters almost always qualified for the belittling treatment, but a freelance reporter who all but guaranteed his story about Rachel would appear on the front page of the Australian was another matter. She had rung the Australian newspaper and received so guarded a reply it convinced her Hunt might be telling the truth. She rang him back.

"Could he come and interview Ms. Demarra on Monday evening?" he had asked.

No, she was out at an important meeting with Fox Studios regarding a new movie.

"Later on that night?" Hunt had suggested.

No, she was attending an après meeting dinner. A possibility existed on Tuesday afternoon, Tuesday morning was out. Chikkie knew Rachel would probably need to sleep off the booze up on Monday night. Tuesday evening would be satisfactory, provided Mr. Hunt took her to dinner at a suitable restaurant. She would supply a short list. The rest of the week was completely impossible, then they were flying back to the States.

Hunt asked for the list to be sent to his email address, and said he would arrive at her suite at seven thirty on Tuesday evening.

"No," Chikkie ordered, "you will wait in the foyer from six p.m. onwards at Ms. Demarra's convenience. Ask the concierge to inform me when you get there."

That way, Chikkie thought to herself, *I can check him out.* If he's a real hunk, Rachel would want to know in advance so she could select an appropriately seductive evening dress.

Hunt pocketed his badly scratched mobile phone and smiled at the others in the room.

"Monday night," he said. "Game on."

The black stretch limousine drew to a halt opposite the Sydney Hilton's ornate glass foyer doors. The valet went forward, and opened the rear door with a small bow. Rachel Demarra stepped out a little unsteadily, and without so much as a nod or a thank you, propelled herself towards the entrance. A uniformed porter opened the door as she staggered inside, noting, as she passed, the definite aroma of Bourbon. The woman was as tight as a drum. Ms. Demarra made her way over to a young valet standing not far from the central check-in desk. He straightened up as he saw her approach. Surely the film star wasn't coming over to speak to him? She was. His evening was made.

He bowed slightly. "Ms. Demarra, can I assist you in some manner?"

Ms. Demarra came right up close. She seemed younger than he had previously thought, and very beautiful. No wonder men were always falling at her feet. He could feel a dampness spreading under his collar.

"You can." She smiled at him. "What's your name?"

She came even closer. This was an evening his mates were going to hear about.

"Err... George, Ms. Demarra. George Hammond."

"George," Ms. Demarra purred, batting bedroom eyes in his face. "I've forgotten to take my key with me. Such a nuisance. Would you be able to let me into my room? Very discretely, George. There are people watching me all the time, and I wouldn't like anyone else to think I've been so stupid."

"Of course, Ms. Demarra. Shall we take the lift? No, it's down the other side of the foyer. May I help you?"

The stunning Ms. Demarra smelt strongly of Bourbon. So she was a little under the weather, who cared? Once around the corner and safely in the lift, Ms. Demarra steadied herself on George's arm. Sweat broke out on his forehead.

"George, I can call you George, can't I? Can I trust you with a secret, George?"

"Of course, Ms. Demarra, anything."

She reached out a finger and stroked him under the chin. Her touch was gentle, soft, sensuous. George felt a thrill of erotic pleasure course through his body.

"George," she said sweetly, "I have a friend coming up to see me this evening. He is supposed to be somewhere else. I'm supposed to be somewhere else. We would like to be together instead, George. You understand what I mean by together?"

"I... I think I do Ms.—"

"Of course you do, George," Ms. Demarra smiled knowingly. "I'm sure you've been together with a friend many times. Now the thing is, George, I wouldn't like anyone else to know I've arrived, so shall we keep it to ourselves? Oh, and I might step out for a breath of fresh air later, and so if you see me in the foyer again, just pretend our little stroll never happened. Can you do that George? Be my cover man?"

George pledged his silence until all hell froze over. He took out his passkey, swiped it through the reader, and opened the door into Rachel's suite. He felt her caress his cheek as she walked past him, then he shut the door behind her. He touched his cheek where her soft hand had been. She was so hot. Some women were born to remain beautiful all their lives. George made his way discreetly down to the foyer again, his heart still beating fast.

Safely inside her luxury suite, Ms. Demarra removed her coat, wrinkled her nose up at the smell of the Bourbon which had spilled on the collar, and dropped it carelessly on the floor, kicking it under the king sized bed. The smell disappeared. Much better, she thought.

An hour later, George, whose mind was still picturing lovers rolling around in the presidential suite upstairs, noticed Ms. Demarra striding across the foyer towards the lifts again. So she had stepped out like she said. George smiled to himself. Tomorrow night he would be on the same shift. Perhaps there was a chance...

Rachel swiped her passkey through the reader, flew into the bathroom, shedding her clothes as she did. A short time later she emerged totally naked. Walking over to the bed, she threw herself into it and turned off the light, drawing the sheets up around her chin. Soon she was breathing heavily. George would have been very disappointed.

A ghostly figure, with a diaphanous white aura around its form, emerged from behind the heavy curtain and moved silently towards the bed. It spoke loudly.

"Hello, Mother."

Rachel quivered into consciousness. She turned round, took one look at the figure near the window and gave a shriek you could have heard on the harbour. She pressed herself against the bed head as though she was trying to escape through the wall.

"F... FF...FFF... Felicity!"

Rachel drew the sheets up over her naked bosom with shaking arms, unmitigated horror all over her face. The spectre slid closer.

"Stay away from me." Stay away," Rachel screamed again.

"Stay away from you, Mother?" The spectre answered in a soft menacing voice. "After all this time? How many years has it been since you sold my living body to a butcher's pleasures?"

"Wh... wh... what are you here for? Why have you come?" Rachel cried out in terror.

"Can't you guess? Oh, how I've longed for this moment. My pain wracked little body held onto life all those years, while those butchers slowly cut my brain to pieces. But tonight its heart stopped beating, and I was free - to avenge my suffering."

STORM DANCING

"I didn't know. I swear I didn't know," Rachel stammered, horrified.

"Did you arrange my electrocution? You and my ... despicable father?"

"No!" Rachel screeched. "I swear it was an accident. Roger wrecked the lights so we could make love. We had no idea."

The spectre gave a mocking laugh.

Rachel screamed. "It's true. By all that's holy, it's true."

"How much did Ferris pay you for my living body, mother?"

"I couldn't cope. I would have lost everything. You would have destroyed my life. You—"

"How much? I grow tired of waiting. The time of vengeance draws nigh."

A tiny rat-cunning smile flickered across Rachel's terrified face. "You're a ghost. What can a ghost do to me? I turn on the light - you're gone."

The ghost moved closer, its diaphanous white aura rising as it stretched out its arms towards its victim. It laughed. Its victim screamed again.

"Why, mother, how foolish. Imagine, there you are on set, about to use your naked body in the cause of art again. You turn around and there's me. Not like this, oh no, but with my head half off, my eyes gone, my severed brain sticking out, blood running down my poor little face. Somehow I don't think your performance will be up to expectations. How long do you think your wonderful career will last?" The ghostly voice hardened. "Every night, every day I'll be there. Every dream, every waking second until you start to scream and they take you away to a nut house and—"

"Stop. Stop! Alright." Rachel cowered against the bed head. "He gave me a ticket to the States because I'd lost my flight, and a couple of thousand for expenses. He took you away and signed your death certificate. I couldn't cope! You were a vegetable, I—"

"Much better. Now you're going to put that in writing."

The room was suddenly flooded with warm light from the standard lamp near the window. Rachel Demarra stared at the apparition in the nightdress, her eyes dark with disbelief. She looked so solid for a ghost. There was one way to find out. Her right hand shot out and grabbed a pillow, hurled it with all her strength towards the foul spectre. The spectre caught it and hurled it back. The pillow fight ended at that point, however.

The rat-cunning expression returned to Rachel's face. "You're alive. Fancy that. What's all this about, money?"

"No."

"Revenge?" she spat. "You've always ridiculed me, always hated my artistic ability."

"You could pay me no higher compliment, Mother. I don't want your money. I don't want anything to do with you. After tonight I hope I never see your self-serving face again. All I want is my name, the name you stole when you had me declared dead."

"I've a good mind to ring security and get you thrown out," Rachel sneered, and snatched up the phone beside her bed. The fear in her face had been completely replaced with anger. "You've got no proof. I'll tell them I've never seen you before in my life. You can scare the wits out of the other women in gaol."

"Please. Do it," Storm goaded. "You must think I'm totally stupid, mother. Call security and you'll read all about it on the front page of tomorrow's Australian. 'Rachel Demarra sells her injured daughter to be vivisected and experimented on. Shows no remorse, tries to throw her in gaol.' It's all set up. You'll be a household word by tomorrow evening. Famous. Might set your wonderful artistic career back a notch. The public are going to learn all about what happened to me in any case. Whether your name is mentioned or not is up to you."

"You're bluffing."

362

"Care to call my bluff mother? Please, go ahead. Oh, I've been sending our conversation to my friends with this little microphone attached to my mobile phone, and there's a camera in the flower vase over there too. Amazing what they will do in zero light. Black and white, of course, but good enough for any jury I feel."

"You little swine!"

"My friends are on their way now, mother, and you're going to call the desk so they'll have no trouble coming up here." Storm's voice hardened. "One funny move and you're on the front page."

Five minutes later Andrew Craig, Rowland Harris and James Hunt came into the room. There was a lot of paper work and affidavits. Rachel signed them with all the grace of a caged crocodile, occasionally casting reproachful eyes on her daughter to convince herself she was real and to let her know how she felt. If she had known how her daughter felt she wouldn't have bothered. In the end, Rowland gathered everything up into the briefcase he had brought and nodded to the woman on the bed.

"Thank you, Ms. Demarra. We will take our leave."

"What happens now?" Rachel muttered. "When do the police arrive?"

"I don't believe your daughter wishes to press charges," Rowland Harris replied in a very even voice. "Your daughter wishes to change her name in any case, so there will be no public link back to you. I suggest you may wish to contact the insurance company you've defrauded, and come to some arrangement before they notice these affidavits. That is up to you. Good evening."

Andrew collected the crutches he had left outside the door, brought them to Storm, and they all left the room, leaving a stunned Rachel Demarra behind. She wondered what she was going to say to the company who had forked out seven hundred and fifty thousand dollars on a lie. Not for a second did she feel thankful for her own daughter's life. Chikkie Manners was going to have an exceptionally bad day tomorrow.

A very perplexed George, nearly at the end of his shift, noticed Rachel Demarra come out of the lift on crutches, with no less than three other men. What an evening it must have been. His fertile little mind went instantly into overload. A stretch limousine pulled up outside the entrance, and they all disappeared inside.

"How did it go?" Peter asked from behind the wheel.

"Perfectly," Andrew laughed. "Storm was amazing. Rowland has tied everything up. James' plan was brilliant. The woman never knew what hit her."

"I feel bad," Storm said. "I can't even feel sorry for her. You know, she didn't give a damn that I was actually alive and okay, only cared about herself. I hope it won't take very long to change my name, will it Mr. Harris?"

"No, no, not long at all," Rowland chuckled. "You are one remarkable woman, Miss Storm. What a story. I've never enjoyed myself so much for years. Oh, and before we go, you said you'd tell me what you want your new name to be."

Storm fished around in her handbag and extracted an envelope. "It's in there," she said.

CHAPTER 38

Isaac Gilead surveyed the familiar lecture theatre filled with first year medical student hopefuls. All had been admitted to the faculty of Medicine at Sydney University, and would start their studies when the semester began in March. He hated these pre-semester introductions, especially this one. For a week now he had been trying to contact Gerhardt with no success. What had happened to tissue library thirty? Had there been a complication? No one seemed to know anything. Jan Yanac had vanished as well, probably for the same reason. He knew there was some preparatory work to be done, and wished they had taken him into their confidence, even though he wasn't the leader of the project. Now he had been dragooned into doing his usual introduction routine, which, as far as he could see, benefited nobody. The dean, Allan Manning, was winding up his long and laborious introduction. Some of the students in the front row were staring surreptitiously at their smartphones. Now the dean was walking back to his chair.

With a faintly audible sigh Gilead got to his feet, walked to the podium. "May I begin by congratulating you all on your admission to this outstanding university," he began. "I'm sure your presence here is an indication of your excellent academic ability, and your potential to work hard for the accolades which are awarded to this faculty's best."

He paused, recalling to mind the spiel he had delivered so many times before. "You think you have come here to become doctors, but this course is not about making doctors of you. It is about making mechanics. Mechanics skilled enough to repair the most complex, the most astounding machine on the planet, the human body. Within this skin-covered miracle of evolution, you will discover the finest mechanical engineering, the most complex chemical engineering, the most sophisticated electrical engineering, and a level of computer science which makes the very best of our technology seem primitive."

Every face was blank. He sighed, wishing he was back at the research centre. "To become competent mechanics you will learn to think rationally as all good scientists should," he said. "You will learn to make correct and accurate observations, draw reasonable conclusions, and act rationally on those conclusions. You will dispel from your mind any notion that you can repair machines by hope and prayer. You will take full responsibility for your repair work, and not rely on metaphysical magic to make good your incompetence."

Somewhere in the back of the theatre a young woman laughed. It wasn't a cynical laugh, and Gilead checked back over his words to see if he had said anything funny by mistake.

He went on, a small frown wrinkling his brow. "I'm relieved that someone present thinks such notions are laughable. I have recently returned from the United States where a deplorably large number of medical students still hold onto some belief in a god of sorts. Let me tell you now," he thumped the podium with his fist, "such beliefs are dangerous enemies of medicine. When you hand your car over to a mechanic, do you want him to fix it or pray over it?" He cast a critical eye over his audience. "Any doctor who entertains such a belief in God is a menace to medicine, and I will take the greatest of pleasure in eradicating such nonsense. I am aware Australians are far less likely—"

"Oh Professor, I know you're an incredibly gifted neurologist, the world's finest, but you're not God's undertaker. You can't stop people following Jesus."

It was the same joyful voice. The words contained no hint of argument, no trace of offence. Gilead was speechless. Most religious students were defensive or afraid, this one was obviously neither.

He scanned the ranks of seats attempting to identify the speaker. "I take it you yourself are a follower of this mythical person?" he asked.

Once again the laughter, neither mocking nor patronising. Somewhere out there was a student who from the depth of her being, obviously regarded her faith as beyond question. "Of course I am," she answered. "Do you think I'd be stupid enough to follow a dead hero? Dear Professor, I'm not so naïve."

"I'm astounded by your confidence, young woman," Gilead said. "I don't suppose you would care to come forward so we could discuss the issue, right here and now? I warn you, I am no stranger to such debate, and up to this present time I feel I should tell you have never been defeated."

"I feel so sorry for you, Professor. You know so much about the brain, more than anyone, but you cannot discern within its extraordinary complexity the hand of the One who authored it."

Gilead's eyes scanned the back rows of students frantically, searching for the speaker. Somewhere in the third row, he thought, making a mental note to visit his optometrist at the first available occasion.

"Very well," he said stiffly, "please come down and identify yourself. I must say, you have more courage than any student I have so far encountered. I'm sure the dean will not mind if we spend a few minutes clarifying the nature of reality."

The dean glanced nervously at Gilead, but made no move to interfere. From the second back row a young woman was rising from her seat, gathering her crutches, and moving past the other students in the row. He couldn't discern her face from this distance. Now she was in the aisle, making her way down towards him, now he could make out...

Suddenly his face turned ashen grey. His hands began to shake violently. He grasped the podium, his eyes riveted on the approaching figure. His breath was coming in short sharp gasps, his mouth open, frozen in shock and disbelief. Closer now, there could be no mistake. He stared into those beautiful brown eyes, eyes which even now held no malice, only sorrow for his disbelief. The words which fell from his dry lips were hardly audible.

"Odette. My Odette. What have they done?"

She was at the bottom of the theatre now, directly in front of him. She stopped.

"Remember me, professor?" she said, quietly.

Her words exploded in his ears.

She turned and made her way out of the theatre on her crutches, leaving Gilead clutching the podium to prevent himself from falling, staring after her in sheer disbelief. Around him the sound of astonished voices began to rise, murmurs of "What happened?" "Who was that girl?" "Look at Gilead. He's seen a ghost."

The Dean leapt from his chair. "Isaac, what's the matter? You're ill, allow me to help you."

He turned to the astonished audience. "Professor Gilead is unwell. This introduction will conclude. Thank you for your attendance. Please allow me to escort Professor Gilead to medical assistance before you leave."

Taking Gilead by the arm he made his way towards the exit. Just before he arrived there, another man who had been seated in the front row, rose and barred their path.

"Professor Gilead," the stranger said, "my name is James Hunt from the Australian. Tomorrow morning the paper is running a story which alleges that you, Professor Gerhardt Metzger and a number of others took a living human being, reported her as dead, and for two and a half years, without ethical approval of any sort, conducted experiments on her brain. This young woman escaped a final attempt to have her murdered. Several weeks ago, learning that she was still alive, you tried to re-acquire her as tissue library thirty, amputate her limbs and continue your experiments. I wonder if you have any comment?"

Gilead froze aghast. Betrayed, doubly betrayed.

He answered quietly. "I have nothing to say, except this. Tomorrow you will destroy one of the greatest achievements of medical research, as well as the great minds who brought it about. You should feel proud."

With that he walked away, detaching his arm from the Dean who looked as though someone had just removed his kidneys without asking him first. Over in the far distance a girl stood, her arms wrapped around a young man's neck, her crutches in his hand.

CHAPTER 39

That night there was a celebration in the Craig's house which all those present would remember for the rest of their lives. A number of very special guests had been invited, Matthew, from the Supermarket, Annette, Andrew's secretary, Daniel Lucas, Rowland Harris and James Hunt. Even police commissioner Robin Naylor had asked if he could attend, so Detective Inspector Ray Wright had to come along as well. He was glad he did.

The superb food had arrived at the hands of some expensive caterers, ordered and paid for by Rowland who would brook no opposition. The fine wine had been provided by the Australian newspaper itself. After the meal, James Hunt, assisted by Andrew and Brian, recounted the story which would appear in the morning's edition, watching the eyes of those not in the know grow larger and larger in the telling. James never took his eyes off Storm the whole evening, something Peter, a picture of misery on the edge of the crowd, never failed to notice.

When all had been told, Storm stood up with her glass in her hand. "I want to thank you all," she said. "It seems such an inadequate word. I owe my life to so many of you. Uncle Brian and his friend Daniel saved me from drowning. If it wasn't for Uncle Brian and the police, I'd still be afraid of being recaptured and destroyed. I want to thank Matthew for his incredible kindness to an unknown artist."

"Mr. Harris has been so generous in dealing with my complicated and sordid affairs," Storm continued. "James, you saved me from being butchered. I can never thank you enough."

She gave him one of her loveliest smiles. Peter winced.

"Without you I'd be dead," Storm continued. "I owe you my life. But most of all I want to say thank you to my wonderful family. Darling Ellen, my brilliant little sister, you saved my life too. If it wasn't for you I wouldn't have a family at all. Not only did you save me, you gave me my beautiful name, Storm. I love you so much, Ellen. Peter, my wonderful brother, who cares for me far more than his own heart. Then Mum and Dad. You took me in, a damaged girl without a name, without a past, when all I did was upset your breakfast and pee all over your floor. You gave me a home. You taught me... loved me. I can't tell you how much I love you all in return. I'm so blessed. God has been so, so good to me. No one else can say they've been born again twice, but I have." She raised her glass. "To my wonderful family," she said.

Everyone in the room was cheering, clapping. Andrew and Basa folded her into their arms.

Andrew, his arm still around Storm's shoulder, turned to the audience. "Storm, no family could be more proud of you, no family could love you more. Ladies and gentlemen, here is a young woman of exceptional, extraordinary courage and faith. She came to us a few years ago without words, without knowledge, without a past, but with a beautiful heart. It is we who have been blessed, Storm. Your warmth, your love, your determination, have been an inspiration to us and to all who have come to know you." He raised his glass. "To our daughter Storm," he said.

The cheer could have been heard down the street. Ellen threw her arms around Storm's waist, holding on for a long time and saying nothing at all. Peter moved near and rubbed her shoulder.

"You're an angel," he said quietly. "A beautiful, brilliant angel."

"So," Ellen said, detaching herself at last. "Isn't it time we knew your proper name? You've been keeping it a secret long enough."

Storm laughed, and walking unsteadily over to the kitchen, extracted an envelope from the top drawer and made her way back with slow, deliberate steps.

"It's thanks to Mr. Harris," she said, "and it's official. I have a new name." She handed the envelope to Ellen. "Tell them."

Ellen tore open the envelope, read the contents and exclaimed in an astonished voice. "Storm *Dancing*? Not Craig? Why? You're a cripple, not a dancer."

Storm laughed. "Yes, I am, but my heart dances all the time. I'd so much rather be a cripple with a dancing heart than a dancer with a crippled one."

There was an explosion of laughter, followed by applause from all. Peter, unnoticed by anyone except Storm, quietly withdrew down the corridor and went into his room.

Within half an hour of this joyful announcement, all the guests had departed.

James was the last to leave. "When all this is over, Storm, would you mind if we had dinner together or something?" he asked.

She gave him a beautiful smile, threw her arms around his neck and kissed him on the cheek. "That would be nice. Thank you, James. I'll never forget you."

"I don't want you to forget me. I'd like you to get to know me a bit better."

She smiled. "We'll see," she said.

There was hardly any washing up to do, the caterers had taken care of all that, and in a short time the house was ready to face the next day. Storm took the last collection of glasses into the kitchen and stowed them in the dishwasher. She turned round to find Andrew standing close to her.

STORM DANCING

There was a strange expression on his face. He placed his hands softly on her shoulders, and Storm returned his gaze with big, brown, speaking eyes.

"Well, young lady, so it's Storm Dancing, is it?" he said, quietly. "I always thought you wanted to be a Craig."

"A girl has to have a name of her own before she can give it away."

"I thought as much," he sighed. "My son believes you're falling head over heels for James Hunt."

"But you know I'm not, don't you, Daddy?"

"I do. Dear Peter, so very clever in many things, can't see what's plain before his face. I think you'd better tell him, don't you? Before he goes into a complete decline."

"You approve, Daddy?" Storm asked with large, sparkling eyes.

"My darling Storm, how could you doubt it?" He hugged her tight, gave her a final kiss on the cheek. "I'm going to bed. Basa is waiting. Goodnight, Storm Dancing."

"Goodnight Daddy."

Storm went down the hallway on her crutches and into her bedroom. What to wear? She glanced at the dressing gown hanging up on the door and decided no. She was a follower of the Way, and there was no point in making her desire harder to control. Out of her cupboard she selected a Desigual top, one which showed just the right amount of cleavage, and put it on. Jeans? No, a skirt. She dropped them to the floor and selected a blue one, edged with small white flowers. She sat down at the dressing table, and brushed her hair into perfection. Makeup? Yes, a little. She highlighted her eyebrows in dark brown. Good, then a soft shade of lipstick, not too much, perfect. Now just the right amount of perfume, she knew which one. Shoes? No, bare feet. She considered using her crutches, decided this was not the time, and walked unsteadily out across the corridor.

She knocked on Peter's door. "Can the distraction come in?"

A grunt was all she received in reply. Good enough, he wasn't asleep, which had been her main worry. She entered the room. Peter was sitting on the side of his bed, looking as though the world was about to end. He turned round at the sound of the door opening. The mournful expression on his face morphed into quite another, and Storm, watching the change, glowed with satisfaction. Peter's mouth was half open in astonishment.

To his eyes her whole body seemed to shimmer with a secret delight. Her eyes bright and beautiful radiated a suppressed joy, ready to explode. Her perfect breasts thrust out the colourful soft material of her top in a mesmerising curve, which moved gently with every step she took towards him. The blue skirt – the one Peter really loved her wearing – swished gently around her knees in a most beguiling manner. Now she was closer the fragrance of her perfume wafted around him, conjuring visions of her body warm and eager against his own, her lips pressed passionately against his kiss, her arms around his neck.

He shut his eyes and groaned. She had probably just spent the last thirty minutes doing that with James Hunt. The complete stupidity of the thought never crossed his mind for a second. Somehow he knew this was the end. He couldn't go on this way anymore. To tell her meant he would lose her forever. Well, he had lost her anyway. Life had descended into a cruel farce.

He never meant to say the words, yet somehow they escaped his mouth before he could recall them. "Oh Storm, you're so... so ... beautiful."

"Why so sad, Peter? Hasn't it been a wonderful evening?"

The moment of truth had come. Peter threw out his hands in front of him in a gesture of total despair, and slapped them down on his knees. "It's no good, Storm. I can't do it. The whole thing's become a farce. I can't be your brother anymore."

Storm Dancing

Storm arranged her face into just the correct proportion of shock and concern. "Peter, why ever not?"

Peter filled his eyes with the beautiful creature who was now sitting next to him, and slapped his knees hard again. "No, no! You don't understand. I love you, Storm."

"Of course, Peter. I've known that forever. I love you too."

"No, you don't understand at all." Peter shook his head miserably. "I'm IN love with you, Storm. I adore you. I started to fall in love with you the day you came to breakfast, and it's been growing ever since. I want to hold you in my arms. I want to kiss you, make love with you, have children with you, and be your lover and protector every day for the rest of my life. I want to wake up and watch your eyes open beside me. If I can't do that my life isn't worth living. Now you know."

She reached out her hand and placed it softly over his. "Of course, Peter. I've known that forever."

He stared at her, totally stunned and uncomprehending. "W... what? Then if ... does that—"

Storm turned suddenly, and with her right hand pushed hard against his chest. He fell backwards onto the bed, his legs dangling over the edge. In a smooth movement she rolled her body right on top of him. Holding his arms down against the doona with her hands, she covered his mouth with her warm, soft lips in a long, passionate, and most un-sisterly kiss. Beneath her breast she felt his heart surge to the same fierce beating as her own. Finally she lifted her head up, close to his own incredulous face.

"And now," she said breathlessly, "what was that ridiculous question you wanted to ask?"

CHAPTER 40

Storm Dancing married Peter Craig before the year had run its course, and although both of them still live with the Craigs, there couldn't be a happier, closer family. Ellen knocks before she comes into their bedroom, the only change her brother and sister (in law) absolutely insisted on.

The Australian ran the story for a whole week on the front page under the by-line of James Hunt, freelance reporter now working for the paper, and followed the court cases when they occurred over the year. Of the doctors who were involved with the project, Ross, who assisted the prosecution, was struck off from further medical practice for twelve months. Festerhaus had disappeared, Hargraves, now resident in the USA could not be extradited for some reason. Gilead, Metzger and Yanac were struck off permanently and all received gaol sentences. Gilead's was reduced on account of the strong plea made on his behalf by Storm Dancing through her Barrister, Rowland Harris. The support staff received various censures, all except Pat Fletcher who had turned evidence for the prosecution. ARG washed their hands of the whole matter, claiming they had not been informed, and up to this time the procedures used by the team to successfully grow frontal cortex have not been released, much to the detriment of medical science which also lost some of its finest minds.

Storm Dancing

Isaac Gilead is serving his gaol sentence in a low security facility near Sydney. Rejected by his colleagues and the academic community and bereft of friends, he has only one constant visitor who often comes with her husband. Sometimes they talk about neurology, which is very helpful to the young lady, who is on the dean's honour's list each year in her medical degree, but most of the time they talk about God.

The End

MAC CUSITER

ABOUT THE AUTHOR

Mac Cusiter was born at Lewisham, a suburb of Sydney. His boyhood interest in science culminated in his graduating from Sydney University with a doctorate in physical organic chemistry. He began his professional life as a Chemistry teacher at Sydney Institute, and retired as head of the science department. He has been a youth leader for much of his life, and is at present a pastor at Christ Church Northern Beaches.

He lives with his wife Val in Sydney's northern suburbs.

Also by the author

THE BREACH

Doctor Daniel Van Dekker is a worried man. Political engineering destroyed Australia's world class Institute for Nuclear Research. As chief scientist he had failed to protect the institute he loved. Furious with his political masters and angry with himself, Dekker pressured the government to allow him to conduct experiments into nuclear fusion, holding out the promise of cheap energy and intellectual property rights worth a fortune. To this his political masters agreed, their hidden agenda to ensure Dekker's failure and subsequent humiliation.

But Dekker also had a hidden agenda

Instead of investigating nuclear fusion he planned to perform high energy collision experiments with the aim of discovering new fundamental particles,

If he was successful, Australia's reputation in nuclear research would be restored.

But Dekker's experiment went horribly wrong.

With only two scientists on his team, Dr. Mark Chambers, a particle physicist and a committed Christian, and Dr. Candice LeBlanc, a power engineer who hates religion of any sort, Dekker must solve the problem he has created.

He has just had to flee the country to save his life.

www.ingramcontent.com/pod-product-compliance
Lightning Source LLC
Chambersburg PA
CBHW071201250626
47159CB00001B/164

* 9 780099 415815 *